Eight Shifts for Wellness

by Marc Levin

"Since my MS diagnosis 11 years ago, health and wellness has become of utmost importance to me. Marc Levin's *Eight Shifts for Wellness* is a practical guide that helps to adjust the reader's common views of wellness and put them into perspective. He asserts that wellness is a frame of mind in which one should always be striving to improve, making choices in your best interest, and maintaining a well balanced lifestyle."

~Montel Williams, author of *Living Well: 21 Days to Transform Your Life, Supercharge Your Health, and Feel Spectacular*

"Life is a series of shifts and adjustments to change! In his book *Eight Shifts for Wellness*, Marc Levin has provided us with the tools necessary to make those shifts to point our lives in the right direction."

~Wayne B. Jonas, M.D., president and CEO of the Samueli Institute and former director of the Office of Alternative Medicine of the National Institutes of Health

"Marc Levin illuminates an issue at the core of personal health and wellness. These Eight Shifts will move readers from the stage of having a "good idea about," to the stage of "making a dynamic choice." This book is about ownership of and responsible participation in all aspects of life, i.e. wellness! Every health practitioner would do well to write every client a prescription for this book."

~Regina Sara Ryan, author of *Wellness Workbook* (with John W. Travis, M.D.), and *After Surgery, Illness or Trauma*

"Marc Levin has written a very valuable, very helpful, and very readable book. I recommend it highly for anyone seeking an approach to wellness and fulfillment based on wholeness, integration, personal choice, and empowerment. Incorporating the best of Eastern wisdom, individual intuition, and a context in which Western medicine can be most appropriately included. *Eight Shifts for Wellness* is a roadmap for sustainable wellness. It lays out in clear terms the primary changes or shifts in mind-set and behavior that lead to lasting well-being in our lives. Read it, share it, and most importantly, apply it in your life."

~Chalmers Brothers, author of *Language and the Pursuit of Happiness: A new Foundation for Designing Your Life, Your Relationships and Your Results*

"Marc Levin's business background gives him a uniquely practical perspective as he offers eight strategies for living a fuller, healthier, and more satisfying life."

~John G. Sullivan, Ph.D., author of *The Fourfold Path to Wholeness: A Compass for the Heart* and *Living Large: Transformative Work at the Intersection of Ethics and Spirituality*

Eight Shifts for Wellness

Practical Transformative Steps to Enhance Health, Wellness, and Well-Being

Marc Levin

GOLDEN NUGGETS PRESS

Golden Nuggets Press, LLC
P.O. Box 351
Fulton, MD 20759
www.GOLDENNUGGETSPRESS.COM

For information about special discounts for bulk purchases, please contact the publisher via mail or info@GoldenNuggetsPress.com.

ISBN: 978-0-9832828-0-8
Library of Congress control number: 2011920833

For Kim, Jason, Megan, Alex, Jake, and Peggy.

Knowledge and wisdom for the sake of others.

Contents

Preface

～

B efore you delve into the meat of this book, it may be useful for you to understand how and why it came to be written. In 1975 a small healing arts clinic was founded in Maryland and has since grown and blossomed into the Tai Sophia Institute, a unique accredited graduate school focused on health and wellness. For over thirty years there has been an expanding conversation about health and wellness taking place among the Tai Sophia (pronounced tie so-fee-a) community which includes a reframing of how these concepts can be viewed in a way that better serves us all.

As life would have it, a number of years ago I happened to have the good fortune to begin working at the Tai Sophia Institute in the accounting and finance department. I am a certified public accountant with an MBA. At the time I began my employment at Tai Sophia I was not particularly knowledgeable about or interested in health and wellness topics. I had very limited awareness of practices, modalities, and philosophies in these areas beyond those of the traditional Western model and was not inclined to read books or articles about them. You could say I was a fairly average guy working hard to provide for his family but not actively pursuing any type of personal growth or rediscovery of the meaning of life or of why I might want to change my attitude toward my health and wellness.

My experience with the Tai Sophia Institute changed all of that and provided the genesis for this book. As a new employee I noticed that the staff, founders, faculty, and students spoke about life, health, relationships, and work differently than I had experienced elsewhere. It was clear to me from these early experiences that I had stumbled into a very unique place and had an opportunity to learn many things of value. I began attending community programs and classes, read articles, and earned a graduate certificate in transformative leadership. I am now in the final stages of earning a master's degree in Transformative Leadership and Social Change from Tai Sophia. What struck me about what I was hearing and learning and being exposed to was that it all made logical sense. This wasn't new-age thinking or fringe concepts. It was reasonable knowledge and wisdom that was grounded and practical.

The fundamental principles, concepts, and distinctions that I encountered at Tai Sophia were the inspiration that led me to conduct additional research on health and wellness. I conceived and wrote *Eight Shifts for Wellness* because I believe that it will serve others, as it has served me, to be exposed to powerful new possibilities in addressing health and wellness issues. It contains my interpretation, perspective, and research on these topics and I am not speaking on behalf of the Tai Sophia Institute. The book contains both material taught there and material not taught there.

My approach to communicating the information and concepts you will find here is one of presenting what I call "golden nuggets in a nutshell." As a result of my financial training I tend to be analytical and strive to home in on the key information and what it means relevant to any topic. For the topics covered in *Eight Shifts*, I succinctly provide you—"in a nutshell"—with valuable background information, including the logic behind the application of that information, while highlighting the "golden nugget" that you can put to practical, immediate use. I aim to share and explain the material in a useful, logical, understandable, and perhaps unique way because of my passion for the power and potential it has to change your life, the lives of your loved ones, and the lives of others.

Introduction

⤳

You have the power to impact your own health. You have the power to impact your own wellness. You have the power to impact your own well-being. You have the power to choose how to deal with any situation. You have the power to take control of your life. You have the power to impact others' health and wellness. You have the power to impact the wellness of the world.

Eight Shifts for Wellness contains concepts, information, activities, skills, distinctions, and practices that you can use to impact your health and wellness and improve your life and the lives of others. It suggests a new way of looking at and new possibilities for relating to your own health and wellness. It offers a practical common-sense approach to addressing health and wellness issues and provides concise, logical explanations in support of the concepts. It describes and illustrates eight shifts each of us can make in how we think and act and live in order to enhance our own and others' health, wellness, and well-being.

The actions we take, the choices we make, the way we think, the way we act or react to situations, the way we move through life all impact our health and wellness more than we may realize. The concepts and information and principles covered in this book are powerful and universal. They apply regardless of what country or city you live in, what religion you subscribe to, what your economic situation is, what age you are, what your political point of view is, what language you speak, or which gender you belong to. I believe that the concepts and information you will encounter here are so fundamental that if the book were randomly given to one hundred strangers in any city, town, or village in the world each of them could use the material to make a positive impact on their health, wellness, and well-being. Though each person may find different concepts or practices that he or she connects with and chooses to apply, everyone would find at least one idea, concept, or practice that would touch and benefit them.

It can be argued that we tend to live our life and make decisions based on our default settings. Making a change requires some effort and some assistance, but it can be done. Each of us is capable of improving our health and wellness by shifting out of our default settings and transforming how we live our lives. Transformations can occur by awakening to new ways of looking at or relating to something, whether it be a general life issue or a specific problem: a health concern, a relationship, a challenging circumstance. Transformations can occur by looking at the world differently and seeing new possibilities, new opportunities, and new choices.

One model for experiencing a transformation is to move through a process or cycle in which you first look at a subject such as health and wellness with a fresh new perspective you did not previously consider. You increase your awareness and reframe how you view the issue. Next, you become aware of and informed about new possibilities for addressing the issue; you begin to consider new choices, options, alternatives, and opportunities. At that point a meaningful shift takes place where you change your way of thinking and acting and the choices you make.

A transformation occurs when you embody the new learning and repeatedly shift your way of thinking and acting, which results in a fundamental change in your actions and approach to life.

The goal of this book is to be a catalyst for change by providing you with the information, knowledge and background that will enable you to move through this process for the sake of yourself, your loved ones, and future generations. You will be exposed to new possibilities for impacting health and wellness and for living life from a different context. You will have an opportunity to shift not only how you think about health and wellness but to act in support of your newfound understanding. Practices will be suggested that can assist you in embodying the new learning so it can be integrated into your daily life.

The inspiration and foundation for this book is rooted in the teachings, philosophy, values, practices, and themes I became exposed to at Tai Sophia, whose wellness-based studies are anchored in the modern world while respecting ancient wisdoms.[1] The information and concepts in *Eight Shifts* are based on fundamental principles and practices that have been used successfully by many different cultures and peoples from all over the world. The book is not about good or bad, right or wrong, Western medicine vs Eastern medicine, or traditional vs complementary modalities. It is about exposing you to some ways of looking at health and wellness that you may not have considered before. It is about introducing you to practical concepts and ideas and creating a wider array of options that are available to you as you move through the dance of life. It is about creating an opening for you to make powerful shifts that will serve you and those with whom you interact.

Imagine yourself sitting with family and friends at a popular restaurant called Fusion. Though you're not familiar with the food they serve, you're willing to give the restaurant a try because it was highly recommended. When the waiter comes to your table, you ask him to tell you about the restaurant. He says, "We specialize in fusion cuisine which combines elements of various traditions from different countries and cultures from around the world. The blending of spices, flavors, and ingredients from multiple cultures results in a unique dining adventure."

The waiter then leaves to give you some time to look at the menu. You see some items that you've never heard of as well as some familiar-sounding dishes that you suspect may taste different at this restaurant. When the waiter returns you ask him to make a recommendation about what to order. He informs your group that the chef suggests a specially designed four-course dinner that introduces new patrons to the restaurant's style of cooking and its benefits. He explains that the four courses—soup, salad, main course, and dessert—as well as the specific items in each course are selected to complement and build upon one another to create a powerful dining experience.

The waiter continues to describe the specifics of how that dining experience is created. "One unconventional feature of this restaurant is that we use the term 'shift' rather than 'item' or 'dish,'" he tells your party. The soup is a shift called *reframing* and establishes the base from which to introduce your taste buds to something other than traditional cooking. The salad course is next, for which the chef has prepared a delicious shift she calls *empowerment* that builds on the flavors of the soup and prepares you to savor the main course. The main course is comprised of four tasty shifts the chef calls *awakening, choices, living,* and *possibilities.* These shifts launch you into the world of fusion cooking with its bountiful rewards and delicious nuances. The meal is elegantly capped off with a delectable dessert of two shifts that are in high demand: *partnership* and *service.*

You can think of this book as a four-course meal at Fusion designed to assist you in experiencing a unique approach to wellness. The restaurant analogy can also be used to illustrate potential reactions to the material in the book. Similar to visiting a restaurant for the first time, there is value in trying various dishes and being open to a new way of preparing a meal. You may instantly like some dishes, while your friends prefer others. You may need to taste some dishes more than once to appreciate them because you have grown accustomed to a different style of cooking. If you like what the restaurant has to offer and you enjoyed and benefited from the experience, you will hopefully revisit it frequently and recommend it to your friends.

As you are reading the book, some concepts will have more meaning for you than others. Some will resonate in a special way for you. You may read something and say to yourself that it's obvious or just common sense. Yes, it is. Or you may say, "I knew that," or "I do that sometimes." The key to living it rather than just "knowing" it is to internalize the information and apply the skill or practice frequently and routinely in your daily life.

Just because something appears simple or basic does not reduce its value. Many of the ideas in *Eight Shifts* are based on ancient practices or philosophies that are grounded in wisdom traditions. Some may sound strange or unscientific to you because you are not familiar with them. Many wellness practices used routinely in other parts of the world which may in the past have been considered mysterious, strange, or unscientific are now being accepted in Western society.

Unlike healing practices of the East, the medical system in the United States is based on a disease management model that does not address a person's whole being. Doctors are taught to deal with diseases, not to promote and enhance a patient's wellness. Health insurance is structured to pay for treating diseases, not for providing services to keep you healthy or improve your well-being. There are healing traditions in other parts of the world that reflect a broader view and approach to wellness.

According to the National Center for Health Statistics and the National Health Survey, the typical adult in the United States has seven chronic conditions, and at least 90 million Americans currently live with chronic illnesses. Researchers have estimated that 70 percent of all illnesses, including those that are chronic, can be prevented.[2]

Heart disease, diabetes, prostate cancer, breast cancer and obesity account for 75 percent of health care costs; yet these conditions are largely preventable and even reversible by changes in lifestyle: diet, exercise, response to stress. Chronic pain is one of the major contributors to the cost of workers' compensation claims. Yet there are effective methods for addressing pain other than the prescription and bioscience approach.[3]

Sickness, disease, and medical conditions will not be eliminated. The material in this book will not make anyone disease free or symptom free. It can be used, however, to empower you to take steps to enhance your health and wellness.

Life is constant movement, and we cannot control what it throws at us. What we can control is how we deal with it. We have the power to decide how to act in any situation, and the choices we make have a powerful impact on how well we are and the quality of our life. There are skills and practices we can use to assist us in making those choices.

We all are continually interacting with others—with family, friends, coworkers, community members, and strangers. We have the power to impact their wellness and well-being. We have the power to be a positive influence in their lives. The principles, concepts, and information you will encounter in *Eight Shifts* will assist you in being that influence. As you read the material, think what it would have meant to you and how different your life, health, and wellness might be now if you had been taught these concepts and practices when you were a child. Then envision a future where children are taught them beginning in preschool and elementary school. Envision a future where the college curriculum for students preparing for teaching careers is expanded to include information on health and wellness so our future educators can teach children basic techniques for living a healthier life. Envision a future where the curriculums at nursing and medical schools are expanded to include a broader framework for impacting health and wellness. Envision a future where people are provided easy access to information, training, and support on these concepts.

There is a difference between knowing or learning something and applying it. The concepts, information, bits of wisdom, and suggestions in this book are useless if they are not applied and practiced. Implementing changes in our lives is an active process that necessitates our being engaged in it. Practice needs to show up in the world to have an impact. When we are "in practice," what we do makes a difference in our lives and in the lives of others. For that reason the book includes a chapter listing practices you can apply on a daily basis to embody the learning and anchor the ideas you've been exposed to.

Finally, each chapter concludes with a section called "Reflections" in which you will find teaching stories and quotes to provide you with additional insights and inspiration. Humans have probably been telling stories since we were first able to speak. Stories have been used to pass on history from generation to generation, to entertain, to romanticize adventures, and to explain the unknown. Teaching stories have been used since ancient times to illustrate a point, teach an important lesson, or make the listener think.

A teaching story is like a piece of abstract art. Each person looking at it has his or her own take on it. You may initially have one interpretation and after repeated or prolonged exposure have a different understanding of the piece. The artist may have had one idea in mind but you may be seeing something else. Some people looking at the artwork may only see what is painted on the canvas, while others may find meaning in the blank areas. It may remind one person of something that elicits a totally different reaction from what someone else experiences.

Similarly, a teaching story may impact each of us in widely differing ways. Teaching stories are intended to provoke the listener to think about the life lessons they illustrate. In reading the stories in this book, think about situations in your life that may be relevant to what each story is about. What is the gift you have the opportunity to receive from it? How can the teachings be applied in future situations you may encounter? What does the story communicate about relationships? How does it relate to your own life at home and with relatives? What possibilities does it offer for your work environment? What effect might it have on your interactions with children? How can you use the knowledge and insight you get from the story to have a positive impact on your well-being and the well-being of others?

Quotations are included in the reflections section because some people find them inspiring, enlightening, insightful, or thought provoking. There may be one quote that touches you and elicits a reaction that changes your life in some way. There may be another that challenges your way of looking at something or provides you with a fresh insight that opens up new possibilities for you. There may be a quote you've seen before that in the light of what you're reading in this book now has new meaning for you. There may be one that you can use as inspiration to improve your well-being or the well-being of others.

My hope and intent is that you encounter in the following pages something that resonates with you and inspires you to make a shift. Life is full of new possibilities for each of us. Let's try some out and see what shows up.

Reframing

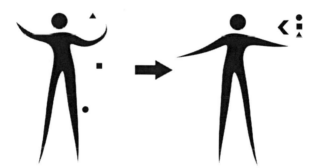

CHAPTER 1

Shift 1: REFRAMING

Shift: View wellness in a context that is much broader than your physical body and within a wellness-based model rather than a disease-based model.

Many people think of health as related only to their physical body: I have a pain, I have an ailment, I have a disease, I am sick, I don't feel well. Wellness is in fact a much broader concept than your physical condition or lack of ailments and is impacted by your mind, your emotions, the choices you make, and how you live your life. Shifting and reframing your understanding of and perspective on health and wellness lays the foundation for making changes to enhance your life.

WELLNESS VS HEALTH

When considering the issue of health, most Westerners think in terms of the presence or absence of disease. Health is perceived as re-lating solely to the physical body and its functions and symptoms. The medical system and approach in Western cultures is based on this view of health and focuses on the treatment of a specific disease or illness.

Wellness is much broader than this common perception of health because it considers all aspects of a person's existence—not just the physical condition but the whole person: mind, body and spirit. Wellness includes one's emotional and psychological as well as physical condition because they are all interrelated.

The World Health Organization defines health as a state of complete physical, mental, and social well-being, not merely the absence of disease or infirmity.[1] The National Wellness Institute characterizes wellness as an active process through which people become more aware of and make choices in support of a more successful existence. It notes that wellness is a conscious, self-directed, and evolving process of achieving full potential that includes a multidimensional and holistic lifestyle.[2]

For our purposes in this book wellness is defined as the constant, conscious pursuit of living life to its fullest potential based on an integrated mind-body-spirit approach that includes healthy lifestyle choices: preventive self-care, natural interventions, regular exercise, sound nutrition, stress management, healthy relationships, and personal development. The term "well-being" is included as a more encompassing concept that includes a spiritual aspect.

The approach to medicine in Western cultures is based on a disease-management system that does not address a person's wellness or well-being. Doctors are taught to deal with diseases, not to consider and foster a person's wellness. Health insurance is based on payments for treating diseases, not on payments for services or products or education to keep you well or improve your wellness.

An important crossroads in the Western view of disease and wellness occurred in the 1800s, when Louis Pasteur, a renowned scientist, put forth the theory that diseases are caused by germs. According to Pasteur's famous "germ theory," there are specific germs that cause specific diseases; these germs enter the body and cause it to become sick. Essentially, the theory implies that germs introduced from outside the body are the key determinant of disease and illness, and the conditions within a person's body are irrelevant.

Western medicine became based on the germ theory, focusing not on the wellness of the patient but on combatting or attacking the disease-causing germ. Consequently, the goal of preventive medicine became not maintaining health but early detection of disease so the pathology or germs could be attacked or negated at an early stage.

Under a system based on this model, the cause of a disease or illness is regarded as external to the person—an extrinsically introduced disease-causing germ—so the individual has little responsibility for his or her own health. Using this model, it is easy to fall into the "It's not my responsibility" trap and tell ourselves: "How I treat my body—what I do or how I live my life—is not a factor in my health because any disease or illness is caused by the nasty outside germ. If I get sick, I can go to a doctor and he or she can 'fix' me by giving me a miracle pill to attack those nasty germs that somehow entered my body. I am not responsible for my own health, or if I can have some impact on it, it's a minor one." Western medicine is based on this model, and in the United States the practice of medicine and decisions about health care policy reflect this disease-based approach.

Another model is that the conditions within our bodies do have a significant impact on health and wellness. For thousands of years Eastern and other world cultures have embraced a model which recognizes that what goes on within our bodies has a major impact on the state of one's health. It reflects that diseases and illness develop from within and that we each have the power to impact our health. Practitioners of health and wellness assist the individual in creating a positive environment within his or her body.

A model or approach to health and wellness based on a belief that the internal conditions within our body is very important recognizes that how we treat our bodies and how we live our lives are key factors. It recognizes the healing power of improving the conditions in the body rather than focusing solely on attacking the disease organism. This model acknowledges that the first step in preventive medicine is maintaining an environment in the body that is conducive to good health.

The distinction between the two approaches is crucial. The model which reflects that our internal conditions are important calls for self-empowerment by taking responsibility for our own health. It results in a partnership between the individual and the health care practitioner in maintaining a state of good health and in addressing illness and disease when they occur. It means that anything we do that alters (positively or negatively) the conditions or environment in our body has an impact on our health and wellness. It means that preventive medicine first begins with taking steps to maintain positive conditions in the body to reduce the likelihood of getting sick. According to this model, there are actions we as individuals can take to promote and protect our own health and wellness without the help of a practitioner if we so choose. It calls for a wellness model rather than a disease-based model.

These two conflicting approaches—the disease model and the whole-person model—offer a fundamental and very important distinction on how we as individuals view our own health and wellness and the actions we take to impact it. If you believe that the internal state of your body has very little effect on whether and to what extent you become ill, then your actions will reflect the belief that the way you live your life has little or no impact on your health. On the other hand, if you believe that what goes on in your body is a major factor in determining whether, how often, and to what degree you become sick, then you realize that your actions and the way you live your life are critical to your health and wellness.

Many cultures and traditions around the world endorse—and have endorsed throughout the ages—the second approach. If this model is correct, it means that each of us can have a powerful impact on improving the state of our health and wellness by changing the conditions and environment within our body.

MIND AND BODY

In a discussion of health, wellness, and well-being, an important concept is the relationship between the mind and the body. There are two primary ways of looking at the mind-body relationship. *Monism* views the mind and body not as distinct entities but as one interrelated system. From a health and wellness standpoint, this approach means that what is going on in your body impacts your mind and emotions, and what is going on in your mind and emotions impacts your physical body. The mind produces changes in the body, and the body produces changes in the mind. Scientific research has proven that a relationship between mind and body exists, and that they impact each other.

The other way of looking at the mind and body is called *dualism*. This model was articulated by Rene Descartes, a French philosopher in the 1600s. According to the dualism model, the mind and body are totally independent entities that do not impact one another. Our emotional and psychological status and our thoughts have no impact on our physical health; similarly, our physical health has no impact on our mind, emotions, thoughts, or mood.

The predominant Western view is that of Descartes: there is a split between the mind and body, with the body viewed as separate and distinct from the mind. The implication of this approach to health and wellness is that you need to treat only the body and the physical symptoms—you do not need to take the whole person into consideration.

Eastern cultures, by contrast, believe that the mind and body are not separate but are related and have an impact on each other. The view of Eastern cultures, Native Americans, and other indigenous cultures throughout the world is to recognize the unity of the whole person. We are not machines composed of totally independent parts. Humans are complex, interrelated wholes with all aspects of our existence impacting other aspects of our being.

From a health and wellness standpoint, the Eastern approach is a whole-person approach because the mind and body are seen as directly related. What goes on in your mind—what you think and how you feel—directly impacts your body, which in turn affects your thinking and emotions. The Eastern model does not deny that external factors can impact disease and illness, but it recognizes that there are internal factors which are equally important. To maintain health and wellness requires treating and considering the entire mind-body complex.

Observe how this relates to you. When you're upset, is there a change in your body? How does it react to your mental state? When you're experiencing stress, what physical changes do you notice in your body? How about when you're excited and happy? In addition to the physical effects you notice, there may be other changes in your various body systems that you're not aware of.

When you exercise, what do you notice about your thinking and emotions? When you've gotten a long night of sound sleep, how does it impact your thinking and emotions? After you take a long deep breath, what changes are you aware of? How does your mood impact your body?

If the monism principle that the mind and body impact one another is correct, you likely notice changes in your body that correlate with what you think and the emotions you experience. Since your mind and emotions impact the conditions in your body and the conditions in your body are a factor in the manifestation of disease and illness, your mind and emotions are a major player in determining your health and wellness.

Similarly, actions you take that impact your physical body, such as exercise or sleep habits, will affect your psychological and emotional state. This is a circular view of health and wellness that contrasts with a linear view in which each aspect of your being is separate and distinct: a tightness in your shoulder is merely a problem with your shoulder that is not related to anything else in your body or life.

Imagine that you're at a local school playground witnessing two children, a boy and a girl, each with a piece of chalk, drawing on the ground. The little girl draws a big circle and stands up at some point on its circumference. The little boy draws a long straight line and stands at the beginning of the line. Then they both begin to walk their drawings. The little girl walks around the entire circle, comes back to her starting point, and continues to walk around the circle. The little boy walks from his starting point to the end of the line and stops.

The little girl walking the circle represents how the wisdom traditions view the natural processes of all aspects of life as a continuous, interacting cycle. The little boy walking the straight line represents how Westerners tend to view the world as separate parts operating in a linear fashion.

Many healing traditions around the world and throughout the ages embrace the circular model of the holistic interrelationship of the mind and the body.

REFLECTIONS

⤳

GOOD LUCK? BAD LUCK?

In ancient times a farmer lived in China with his son. They had an old horse they used to till their fields. One day the horse got loose and escaped into the hills. Each of the villagers came to the farmer to express their sorrow for his misfortune. They said, "What bad luck for you that your horse ran away." The farmer responded, "Bad luck? Good luck? Who knows?"

A few days later the horse returned and was followed by eight wild horses. The villagers came to express their glee and said, "How lucky you are." The farmer responded, "Good luck? Bad luck? Who knows?"

A week later his son was riding one of the wild horses and was thrown to the ground and broke his leg. Once again the villagers came to express their condolences and said, "How unlucky you are that your son broke his leg." The farmer replied, "Bad luck? Good luck? Who knows?"

A few days later the emperor's soldiers came to the village to order all the young men to join the army for an upcoming war. The farmer's son was not taken because he had a broken leg. The villagers came rushing to the farmer to congratulate him that his son was not taken into the army and they told him, "How lucky you are to have such good fortune." The farmer replied, "Good luck? Bad luck? Who knows?"

GOING FOR THE GOLD

There was a man in a village who desired to have gold. He dressed up properly and went out in early morning to the market. He went straight to the gold dealer's shop and snatched the gold away and walked off. The authorities arrested him and questioned him: "Why did you rob them of gold in broad daylight with all the people around?" The man replied, "I only saw the gold. I didn't see any people."³

❧

The beginning is the most important part of the work.

~PLATO

It is the primary role of the physician, whether the African witch doctor or the modern doctor, to entertain the patient while secretly waiting for nature to heal the disease.

~ALBERT SCHWEITZER

There is an Indian proverb that says everyone is a house with four rooms—a physical, a mental, an emotional, and a spiritual. Most of us tend to live in one room most of the time; yet unless we go into every room every day, even if only to keep it aired, we are not complete persons.

~RUMER GODDEN

The significant problems we have cannot be solved at the same level of thinking we were at when we created them.

~ALBERT EINSTEIN

The greatest revolution of our generation is the discovery that human beings, by changing the inner attitudes of their minds, can change the outer aspects of their life.

~WILLIAM JAMES

In the province of the mind, what one believes to

be true either is true or becomes true.

~John Lilly

*All that we are is the result of what we have thought. The
mind is everything. What we think we become.*

~Buddha

*The concept of total wellness recognizes that our every thought, word,
and behavior affects our greater health and well-being. And we, in turn,
are affected not only emotionally but also physically and spiritually.*

~Greg Anderson

*When you are able to get out of the shell of your small self, you will see
that you are interrelated to everyone and everything, that your every
act is linked with the whole of humankind and the whole cosmos. To
keep yourself healthy in body and mind is to be kind to all things.*

~Thich Nhat Hanh

*I see rejection in my skin, worry in my cancers, bitterness
in my aching joints. I failed to take care of my mind,
and so my body now goes to the hospital.*

~Astrid Alauda

The energy of the mind is the essence of life.

~Aristotle

Change your thoughts and you change your world.

~Norman Vincent Peale

*Healthy people are those who live in healthy homes on a healthy diet; in
an environment equally fit for birth, growth, work, healing and dying . . .
Effective health care depends on self-care; this fact is currently heralded as
if it were a discovery. Furthermore, as a Nation, we will spend ourselves*

out of existence in our attempts to prevent suffering and death.
~IVAN ILLICH

The physician who teaches people to sustain health is the superior physician. The physician who waits to treat people until after their health is lost is considered to be inferior. This is like waiting until one's family is starving to plant seeds in the garden.
~YELLOW EMPEROR'S CLASSIC ON INTERNAL MEDICINE, 500 BCE

Things don't change. You change your way of looking, that's all.
~CARLOS CASTANEDA

Empowerment

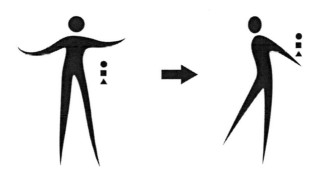

CHAPTER 2

Shift 2: EMPOWERMENT

Shift: You are empowered to dramatically impact your own health and wellness.

As we considered in the last chapter, the state of your health and wellness is not just something that happens to you. You are not an innocent bystander but an active player in determining how healthy and well you are. You are impacting your health and wellness on a day-to-day basis. We all have choices in how we move through and relate to life. If we understand and take personal responsibility for actions that impact our wellness, then we may make different choices. Personal empowerment is accessed through information, knowledge, and self-awareness, not by abdicating responsibility to an outside source or medical practitioner. Shifting to a framework of personal empowerment will lead to an enhancement of your health and wellness.

ROLE OF THE INDIVIDUAL

There are two fundamental principles that have been perennially acknowledged as instrumental in the art of medicine and healing that have been forgotten or overlooked in our modern culture: The individual has a huge part to play in his/her own health and wellness, and the body has a remarkable ability to heal itself.

These principles play a primary role in Eastern medicine, which recognizes that internal factors have an impact on disease and illness and that there are actions which can be taken to promote self-healing. The healing traditions of many indigenous cultures also reflect these principles. These healing traditions incorporate the twin concepts that there is an imbalance in the body which is a factor in the arising of illness and that to treat the illness you must address the imbalance.

It is recognized in these cultures that the individual has a responsibility for maintaining his or her wellness and that his/her actions have an impact on the occurrence and severity of illness and disease processes within the body. Within this model, the healthcare practitioner is not viewed as an expert who is solely responsible for the patient's health. The patient recognizes that the practitioner does not "fix" him or her without his/her actions having an impact. The patient works together with the practitioner as a team to maintain the individual's health and wellness.

In this model, since your unique body and life choices have had a role to play in the illness occurring, no medical practitioner can be expected to "fix" a health problem. The practitioner's actions are designed to enhance your body's ability to heal itself. The relationship between you and the practitioner is critically important because the practitioner is assisting you in healing yourself rather than being an outsider employed to take care of it for you. You could say that healing occurs via relationships: the relationship between you and the health practitioner, the relationship you have with your body, and the relationship between and among your various organs and body processes, all of which you affect, consciously or not.

In cultures based on a wellness model, the role of preventive medicine is to assist you in maintaining your body and life in a balanced state. The focus is on creating conditions in your body such that illness or disease does not occur or that its negative impact is reduced if it does occur. Even Hippocrates, who was responsible for the founding traditions of Western medicine, noted that there are both internal and external causative factors for disease.[1]

Prior to the growth of biomedicine in the 1800s, the physician was viewed as a caretaker who tended and listened to patients in order to nurture them back to health.[2] Physicians and other medical practitioners in the West recognized that the body has the ability to heal itself and provided treatments to promote this healing process. An inside joke in medical circles points to the healing power of our bodies. Insiders say that with a doctor's expert advice you should be better in a week, but without access to the marvels of modern medicine your recovery will require at least seven days.[3]

With the growth of biomedicine, there was a shift in medical doctors' approach to health care. They began to act more like scientists analyzing data and information and placed less focus on caretaking. At the same time, there was a dramatic shift in how patients viewed physicians as they handed off the problem to the doctor and adopted the view that it is his or her job to fix the problem and make them better. Rather than a partnership between the individual and the physician, full responsibility was assigned to the physician.[4]

In addition, rather than feeling a sense of responsibility to maintain their own health, people discounted the impact they have on it, leading to the still prevalent view, "If I get sick it's due to germs from the outside that I encountered and there was nothing I could do to prevent it. It was going to happen and I can just go to the doctor and have him/her give me something to fix it. It's someone else's responsibility to get me better."

In the biomedical model, preventive medicine is regarded as early detection of illness or disease in order to begin addressing it sooner. While early detection is clearly preferred to addressing a disease or illness in its later stages, there is an additional option.

Another viewpoint is that in addition to early detection there are actions we can take to prevent or reduce the occurrence of the disease or illness in the first place. Each of us is empowered to impact our own health and wellness. From an Eastern perspective, anything we do that alters the body's optimal balance (either positively or negatively) has an impact on whether we get sick and to what degree.

If we believe that the conditions within our body play a major role in what effect germs have on us, then anything we do that changes our internal environment has an impact on whether and to what extent we get sick.

CHOOSING EMPOWERMENT

The mind and body are related. The mind impacts the body and the body impacts the mind. The conditions in our body are influenced by our emotions, by what we think, by how we react to stress, by what we internalize, and by how we relate to life in general. Actions we take that change the conditions in our body can have an impact on whether we get sick and to what degree.

This is not to say that illness and disease will not occur and that all illness and diseases can be avoided. It is not to imply a value judgment on Western medicine compared to Eastern approaches. The point is that we can be educated consumers and active participants in determining our own health and wellness and that there may be available to us new possibilities in relation to our health for consideration.

A helpful analogy is to imagine a fire in your house or apartment. If a fire were to start in one room, one approach is to grab a fire extinguisher and put it out before it gets out of hand. This is an early detection model of home preservation that may be effective if you've taken the previous steps of having a working smoke detector and an adequate fire extinguisher available. You would be aware of the problem and be ready to take action before a fire got too big.

Another approach is the prevention model. Using this model you have a fire extinguisher and smoke detector in your house or apartment *and* you take actions to reduce the likelihood of a fire ever starting. For example, you might blow out candles before going to bed, replace frayed or cracked electrical cords, keep flammable items away from the cooking area, keep a screen in front of the fireplace, never overload electrical sockets and extension cords, make sure the stove and oven are turned off appropriately, and run matches under water before discarding them. This is a self-empowerment model in which you take responsibility for practical common-sense actions to create conditions that minimize the risk of a fire and maintain a safe environment in your home. You don't need to have a degree in fire safety to take effective action. You just need to be generally informed and educated on the topic, then implement appropriate behaviors. Taking these steps doesn't guarantee that a fire will never occur, but it will help create conditions that promote a safe home environment that reduces the likelihood of a fire.

Empowerment grows from an awareness that there are actions we can take, choices we can make, and ways we can relate to life that promote our own health, wellness, and well-being. We don't need permission. We don't need a license.

We can reframe our understanding of health and wellness. We can become more self-aware of our body. We can become informed about additional possibilities for addressing our health and wellness concerns. We can shift how we think about them. We can educate ourselves about appropriate actions we can take to impact them in positive ways. Consciously choosing to take those actions is empowerment.

REFLECTIONS

TREASURED POSSESSIONS

Once upon a time in a kingdom far away, there was an unusual custom. In most kingdoms, when the ruler dies, his or her son or daughter succeeds to the throne. But in this kingdom, when the ruler died, a special bird called the "bird of good fortune" was released. The bird would fly around in the air above the subjects in the land and the person upon whose head it finally landed became the next king.

In this kingdom, there was a slave who worked in the palace. He was a musician who entertained the king and his family and guests by dressing in funny clothing—a cap made of chicken feathers and a raggedy belt—and he played music on a drum. The slave was not happy with his lot. He felt that it was degrading, and prayed to be a free man.

It came to pass that one day the king died, and the "bird of good fortune" was released. It circled the sky for some time. All watched in anticipation. Finally it came to rest on the head of the slave, nesting itself in his hat of chicken feathers. Immediately, to his great surprise, the slave was declared ruler of the kingdom. In an instant, the slave was transformed into a powerful sovereign.

The new monarch moved into the palace, donned royal attire, and took his place upon the throne. As his first royal decree, he had a tiny hut built next to the palace. The only furnishing in this little shack was a large mirror. Early every morning, the new king entered this shack, disappearing behind the door for a short time. Then he would emerge, lock the door behind him, and return to the palace. His ministers and advisors thought this was a very peculiar behavior but, after all, he was the king now and who would question the king?

As the years went by, the sovereign passed many laws aimed at reducing and finally eliminating all slavery and much suffering. The changes were made so gradually that no one noticed them. The king was known to all for his kindness, his justice, and his compassion, as well as his strange habit of visiting the odd little hut early every morning.

One day his closest advisor asked, "Your Majesty, what is that you keep in that hut of yours?" The king led the advisor into the hut and showed him a burlap sack, which contained the chicken feather hat, the ragged belt, and the drum. "These," he said, "are my most treasured possessions."

"But these are reminders of slavery!" the advisor replied in disgust. "These are not the possessions of a king, Your Majesty!"

"Ah, but they are," replied the king. "You see, once I was a slave and now I am free. When you made me your king I made a promise to myself. I promised I would never forget that I was once a slave. I feared I would grow arrogant and haughty and treat people as I was once treated. Every morning I come here and dress as I was once forced to dress—as a slave. I stare at myself in the mirror until tears come to my eyes, for only then am I prepared to leave this hut and rule as a good king should. It is this memory that makes me the king I am. It is these rags that are my most treasured possessions."[5]

Patients carry their own doctor inside themselves. We physicians
are at our best when we put that inner doctor to work.
~ALBERT SCHWEITZER

People as a rule find it easier to rely on healers than to
attempt the more difficult task of living wisely.
~RENE DUBOS

To change one's life: Start immediately. Do it flamboyantly. No exceptions.
~WILLIAM JAMES

No one can make you feel inferior without your consent.
~ELEANOR ROOSEVELT

Training began with children who were taught to sit still and enjoy
it. They were taught to use their organs of smell, to look when there
was apparently nothing to see, and to listen when all seemingly
was quiet. A child that cannot sit still is a half-developed child.
~CHIEF STANDING BEAR

What lies behind us and what lies before us are tiny
matters compared to what lies within us.
~RALPH WALDO EMERSON

The curious paradox is that when I accept myself
just as I am, then I can change.
~CARL ROGERS

You create your own universe as you go along.
~WINSTON CHURCHILL

People are like stained glass windows. They sparkle and shine
when the sun is out, but when the darkness sets in, their true

beauty is revealed only if there is light from within.

~ELISABETH KUBLER-ROSS

The person who moves a mountain begins by carrying away small stones.

~CHINESE PROVERB

Whatever you think you can or can't do, you're right.

~HENRY FORD

Awakening

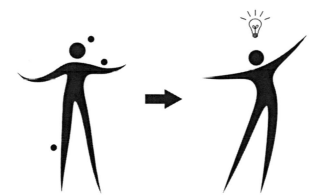

CHAPTER 3

Shift 3: AWAKENING

Shift: Your body is wise.

O ur bodies are innately wise and have much to teach us about restoring and preserving our health if we are willing to listen.[1] A symptom is more than an isolated event. It is a messenger from our body giving us a "heads up." Our symptoms can alert us to an underlying problem that needs attention. We can learn to be better at paying attention and understanding the message that we're being sent. Making a shift to view symptoms as our body's teaching assistants can be an awakening which creates an opening for implementing changes.

YOUR BODY AS TEACHER

Your body is the most brilliant, insightful, caring, nurturing, intuitive, persistent, honest, knowledgeable teacher you have ever encountered. There is much to be learned if you pay attention to it.

Imagine that you're on a beach walking barefoot in the sand and you step on a shell with a jagged edge that cuts your heel. Your foot sends a message to your brain that something has happened, and you feel pain in the foot. You didn't see your foot land on the shell, but because of the pain you're now feeling, you know something happened. You are now in a position to assess the situation and choose what action to take. Perhaps you put a bandage on the cut if you happen to have one with you, perhaps you hop so as not to put pressure on the foot, perhaps you walk with the weight on your toes to reduce the pressure on your heel. Or perhaps you choose to walk normally and just endure the pain from each new step. Because your observer—your mind—was alerted to the injury to your foot, you had the opportunity to choose how to respond to it. If your observer didn't notice the pain, you wouldn't have been aware that you had a cut and would have taken no action. If you took no action, the cut might have become infected and progressed to a major medical condition that would have been avoided by treating the cut when it occurred.

Your body has just functioned as your teacher. It presented you with a situation in which you were free to ignore the pain and suffer the consequences or take appropriate action. You choose what you learn from the lesson.

Your son falls down and scrapes his arm. You wash the scraped area with water and he goes back to playing. The arm starts to repair itself. Over time a scab appears. Gradually the scab becomes smaller and new skin replaces it. Eventually, your son's arm looks the same as it did prior to the fall. Amazingly, the body knows how to heal itself. Most of us don't understand the science of how the body achieves this magical act, but we know that it happens and we accept it.

Your body and mind are interconnected, and they impact each other. When you hurt your foot, your body shares this information with your mind, and you feel pain. When you're worried about something, there is a physical response in your body. When you're excited and happy, your body has a different physiological response.

Some people get sweaty palms when they're nervous. Some get a sharp pain in their shoulders and neck when they feel like they have "the weight of the world" on their shoulders. Some people get headaches when they haven't eaten properly. Some breathe shallowly and quickly when they're anxious about something. These are all examples of your body being a wise teacher and providing you with information that allows you to take appropriate action.

If your observer is alert and you notice the physical phenomena present in your body, you will obtain valuable information that you can use to impact your health and wellness. A pain that you're feeling may be the result of an external incident such as banging your shoulder or cutting your foot; however, if there was not such an event, a physical ailment or change in your body's status could be caused by some internal condition. If you pay attention to your body and address early signs suggesting that something may be wrong, you may be able to prevent larger problems from developing. Addressing these larger, more serious problems may be more painful and costly and may require more invasive interventions.

HEEDING THE "WARNING LIGHTS"

Imagine that you're driving your car and a red indicator light comes on indicating that the car is low on oil. If you don't notice the warning light, you may not know that there is a problem, and the oil level will get lower and lower until eventually the car develops major engine problems which you will then have to deal with. Another possibility is that you see the warning light but put a sticker over it to cover it up so you can ignore it. Since you don't see the warning sign anymore, you assume everything is fine and take no corrective action, but your denial doesn't affect the car's functioning, and the oil level gets lower and lower. Eventually, expensive repairs will be needed to fix the engine. A third option is to pay attention to the red warning light and add oil to the car in response to its signal that oil is needed. This option avoids the more serious and costly problems that will develop if you choose not to address the cause of the problem.

Similarly, our bodies flash "warning lights" in the form of symptoms when something requires attention. If we're not experienced in observing our body and paying attention to it, we may not notice the symptom. Or we may notice it but ignore it or mask it without investigating the message it's sending us. Or we may pay attention to the symptom, take steps to determine the underlying cause, and then take action to address it.

We can learn to become aware of the messages our body is sending us and alert to when something needs addressing. We then have the option of taking action to address the underlying cause.

Think of some symptom that you routinely or periodically notice in your body. These symptoms are the body's teaching assistants alerting you to the need for some kind of action or change. Doing some detective work will help you or a professional evaluate the symptom and the potential underlying cause. For example, notice when the symptom occurs. Does it occur throughout the day or only at certain times? In the morning or evening? When you're sitting, standing, lying? Does it occur every day or only periodically? Do you notice it in conjunction with a particular activity? Is it familiar? Have you had it in the past? Does it move about your body, or is it fixed?

What is your emotional state when you experience the symptom? Are you mad, worried, upset, nervous, anxious or sad? Does it occur during or following a particular situation that appears to precipitate it? Do you experience it more frequently when you're interacting with a particular individual? Does it occur at work, at home, or both?

How long does the symptom last? Is the amount of time consistent? Under what circumstances is the time longer or shorter? What are the circumstances or actions that make the symptom dissipate or disappear? What are your eating habits before it appears? Your sleeping habits? What does it feel like? Is it sharp or dull? Throbbing or persistent? The objective is to gather information and try to isolate the situations and phenomena that surround the symptom's occurrence.

Paying attention to your body may allow you to be much more aware of minor symptoms before they progress to major problems. You may view your body differently and may be more likely to take action before something becomes a serious illness. You may function differently with regard to your pain or illness.

Being healthy does not mean being free from all symptoms. Making the shift to viewing our bodies as wise and our symptoms as teachers or messengers to learn from is an invaluable way to impact our own health and wellness.

REFLECTIONS

⮾

FIGHTING WOLVES

An old Cherokee was telling his granddaughter about a fight that is going on inside each of us. He said it is between two wolves. One is evil: It is anger, envy, jealousy, greed, and arrogance. The other is good: It is peace, love, hope, humility, kindness, and compassion. The granddaughter thought about it for a minute and then asked her grandfather, "Which wolf wins?" The grandfather simply replied, "The one you feed."

THE THIEF

There was a man who had lost money and thought that his neighbor's son had stolen it. He looked at him and it seemed his demeanor was that of a thief; all his gestures and movements were like those of a thief. Soon afterwards he found the money in his house. Again he looked at the neighbor's son and neither his demeanor nor his movement and gestures were those of a thief.[2]

⮾

A bodily disease, which we look upon as whole and entire within itself, may, after all, be but a symptom of some ailment in the spiritual part.
~NATHANIEL HAWTHORNE

We could never learn to be brave and patient
if there were only joy in the world.

~HELEN KELLER

Everything has its beauty, but not everyone sees it.

~CONFUCIUS

The world is a beautiful place to be born if you don't mind
happiness not always being so very much fun, if you don't
mind a touch of hell now and then just when everything is
fine because even in heaven they don't sing all the time.

~LAWRENCE FERLINGHETTI

Health is a blessing that money cannot buy.

~IZAAK WALTON

The part can never be well unless the whole is well.

~PLATO

To view your life as blessed does not require you to deny your
pain. It simply demands a more complicated vision, one in which
a condition or event is not either good or bad but is, rather,
both good and bad, not sequentially but simultaneously. In my
experience, the more such ambivalences you can hold in your
head, the better off you are, intellectually and emotionally.

~NANCY MAIRS

When one is out of touch with oneself, one cannot touch others.

~ANNE MORROW LINDBERGH

Illness is telling us what we need to stop doing. If we look at illness
that way, then it has great value. It might be telling us that we need to
modify our work habits, to rest, or to question what we are doing.

~O. CARL SIMONTON

Choices

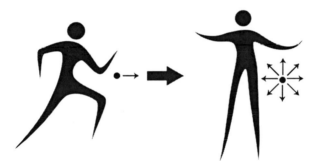

CHAPTER 4

Shift 4: CHOICES

Shift: You have choices in relating to life situations, and those decisions impact your health and wellness and that of others.

Throughout our day we are constantly experiencing life in all of its manifestations. Although there are an infinite number of ways in which we might relate to what we experience, many of us are on automatic pilot. We have learned to relate to life and the situations it presents to us in a certain predictable way. We act or think in a particular manner according to our default setting without being aware of the impact on our health and wellness or the effect our actions have on others. We are not even consciously aware that we have a choice.

We are in fact capable of turning off the automatic pilot and choosing an alternative response that may better serve us. We can each become more awake to the numerous choices available to us in relating to situations and can shift to a new way of being that enhances the health and wellness of ourselves and others.

THE OBSERVER

- Your phone rings and you recognize the incoming phone number as someone you don't want to talk to. You notice that your stomach tightens up and your face gets hot.

- You're talking to a few friends and you notice that one of them has some food caught in her teeth. You think to yourself, "Should I interrupt her and announce that she has food in her teeth? Should I wait for her to finish and pull her aside? Should I point to my teeth as a clue?"

- You haven't been getting your normal amount of sleep this week and you didn't have time to eat lunch today. It's four o'clock in the afternoon and you notice you have a headache and you're having trouble focusing.

- You're in the grocery store doing your shopping and you push your cart into the checkout line. Someone comes up to you yelling that he was about to push his cart into that line and you cut him off. He demands you let him go in front of you. You quickly ask yourself, "How should I deal with this situation? Should I yell back? Should I let him go in front? Should I make believe I didn't hear him? Should I give him a hug and tell him to have a great day?"

- You're talking to your spouse and he/she says something that irritates you. You think to yourself, "Boy, that was irritating. Should I respond to it or just let it slide? If I respond, will he/she get mad and will we get into an argument that will be even more irritating? But if I let it go, he/she won't know that he's/she's wrong."

- You're going about your normal daily activities. You haven't been doing any strenuous activity recently but you notice a tightness and pain in your shoulders.

These situations all have one important element in common. Your "observer" was present. All of us have an observer. Our observer is our ability to notice what is happening in our bodies, in our minds, and in the external situation. Our observer plays a vital role in our ability to control our health, wellness and well-being. In addition to observing our bodies, it allows us to see what is happening, to analyze it, and to make a choice about how to act in response. Our observer allows us to *act* rather than *react*.

Think of the observer as an independent reporter who is giving us data and information without having a vested interest in the situation or the facts. We can then choose what the reported information means to us and what to do with it. We need objective data to make knowledgeable decisions.

We all have an observer within us which we use at different times; however, it is not always present or active. Having our observer in attendance to observe our body is not a skill in which we are practiced. For many of us it requires a conscious effort. You can practice this skill. Close your eyes and observe your body. Describe your breathing. How do your shoulders feel? What is the feeling across your chest? How does your neck feel? Does any area hurt? Is there a sensation in your joints?

By observing your body you can learn a lot that can be used to improve your wellness. Observe your aches and pains. Where does it hurt? How does it hurt? Is it a sharp pain, a throbbing pain, or a dull, persistent pain? How long does the pain last? When does it start? What makes it recede or stop?

Observe not just aches and pains but also general physical conditions: the muscles in your neck tighten up, your leg becomes stiff, your breathing becomes slow and shallow, your face flushes, you clench your fists, you notice a heaviness in your chest.

Observe your physical reaction to specific situations. For example,

- When I skip lunch I get irritable and I'm unable to focus.

- When I'm paying the bills I get a headache.

- When the kids are running around not listening to me my shoulders tighten up.

- When my boss gives me a deadline for a project I start breathing fast and my chest becomes tight.

- When my spouse and I are having a disagreement I get a pain in my stomach.

- Before giving a presentation my palms are sweaty and I feel warm throughout my body. After the speech is over my palms are dry and my body is relaxed.

- After a long walk I notice that my breathing is easier and my body feels lighter.

- When I'm bored in a meeting I sit slouched over, and when I'm interested in what is going on I sit upright and lean forward.

Practice observing your body and describing the feelings and sensations you notice. Most of us aren't practiced at describing our bodies. The following list represents some descriptive words and phrases you might find useful. Feel free to make up words if necessary to accurately portray a mood or sensation.

Tight	Contracted
Closed	Irritable
Open	Tired
Relaxed	Confused
Light	Alert
Hot	Distracted
Warm	Unfocused
Cold	Focused
Flushed	Full
Sweaty	Empty
Knotted	Jittery
Small	Tight
Wide-eyed	Ungrounded
Sleepy	Aching
Sore	Throbbing
Slouchy	Sharp
Rumbly	Dull
Upset	Deep
Elevated	Superficial
Hunched	Intermittent
Knotty	Constant
Prickly	Chronic
Itchy	Persistent
Pleasant	Prolonged
Loose	Jabbing
Stiff	Splitting
Bloated	Pounding
Gnarly	Radiating
Expansive	

You can practice cultivating your observer's skills throughout the day. Your body is continuously giving you feedback. In any situation you can pause to let your observer report to you what is happening in your body. It takes practice but it will prove to be a valuable skill.

You can also practice training your observer to report the facts of a situation in order to allow you to act rather than react. In any situation you encounter throughout the day, pause before speaking or responding. Whatever you're confronting, your observer can be present and report to you in a millisecond. You are already calling upon it throughout the day without even noticing it. When you're driving and the traffic light turns yellow as you approach the intersection, your observer is reporting to you the pros and cons of stopping or continuing through the intersection. You then make a choice.

Imagine watching a movie that's on a DVD or recorded by your DVR. You are emotionally involved in the movie, particularly the current scene. You hit the pause button on the remote. The scene is frozen and you can take a snapshot of what is happening so your observer can report on the facts without all the emotion. You can then evaluate the scene, think about it, consider what may happen next, or reflect on what just happened. Having your observer present is like hitting the pause button on the remote. You get to consider the situation and your actions before the rest of the scene takes place. It creates an opportunity to shift or change your thoughts, emotions, and actions.

Let's look at another example. You're driving down the road with your children and the car in the next lane cuts in front of you, nearly causing an accident, and you yell obscenities at the driver as he's speeding away. Your observer was likely not present and you reacted to the situation. If your observer had been present, you might have evaluated your options with lightning quick speed and chosen a different action than yelling obscenities at a driver who can't hear you. You also might have chosen the same action, but it would have been a choice rather than a reaction.

Calling on your observer more frequently rather than mechanically reacting will require practice and a conscious effort. Like anything else, the more you practice the better you get.

One way to engage or reengage your observer is to focus on your senses. For example, if you find yourself in reaction mode, pause and focus on what you see. Notice the color of your shirt, the shape of the table, the tiles on the floor, the picture on the wall, the ring on your hand. You can focus on what you hear. Notice the blare of the traffic, the background murmur of the radio music, the trill of the birdsong, the hum of the air conditioner. Putting your attention on your sense impressions helps pull the plug on your reactivity and connects the line to your observer.

Having your observer present creates tremendous possibilities. It allows you to make distinctions between phenomena and stories and enables a shift in your thinking. Having choices is empowerment.

PHENOMENA VS STORY

Imagine yourself sitting on a bench in the park. It's a beautiful day and you're enjoying the weather and reading a book. You happen to look up as a man is approaching you along the path. You make eye contact and you note that he looks vaguely familiar. As he looks your way, his expression appears to be questioning. He then starts running down the path. You think to yourself there must be a reason why he looked at you and then started running. He must have recognized you and not wanted to talk to you for some reason so he ran away. You wonder why people think you're unfriendly.

A few days later, you're talking to your mother on the phone. You're having a very nice conversation. Then you tell her that you and your spouse have decided to have another child. There's a pause, and then your mother says she's sorry but she needs to go. She hangs up. You think to yourself that you must have upset her. She must not approve of your decision to have more children. You're annoyed that she didn't even explain why she was mad and just hung up. You wonder if perhaps you should have told her in person. You're angry that she couldn't just be happy for you.

Humans are wonderful storytellers. We love to tell stories. We are very practiced at creating and telling them. We're so good at it that we don't even need to tell our stories out loud. We just tell them to ourselves in our mind. We also like to hold onto a story and keep retelling it.

The two situations above are examples of creating a story. We take facts and create a story around the facts. The story may not be accurate, but that doesn't stop us from telling it. There are an infinite number of stories that can be created around any given set of facts, and we have the power to choose which story we create and tell ourselves.

There is an important distinction between phenomena and story. Phenomena are the physical observations that we notice using our senses. The story is our interpretation of the data and the conclusions we draw about the phenomena. Our interpretation may or may not be accurate.

In the park scenario, the data our observer reports is that a man is walking on the path. His head moves to the right. His eyes appear to move to the right. The muscles on his face appear to tighten, his mouth opens slightly, and his eyebrows curl upward. The man starts running. These are the facts, the physical observations.

The story components are that the person made eye contact and was looking at you. He may have been looking at you or may have been looking over your shoulder at something going on behind you. That he got a "questioning" look on his face is a story you told yourself based on your interpretation of his facial movements. Perhaps he suddenly felt sick to his stomach and the movements of his facial muscles were related to that feeling. Perhaps he was about to sneeze and suppressed it.

The thought that the man recognized you and that was what prompted his running away is a story. He may not have even seen you because he was looking behind you. He may have looked at you but not recognized you. He may have looked at you and thought you looked like someone he knew. He may have looked at you and thought you looked like a movie star.

The fact that the man started to run may have nothing to do with you at all. Perhaps he remembered a forgotten appointment. Maybe he thought of something he needed to do at home. Perhaps he comes to the park every weekend to run and uses the bench you were sitting on as a starting place to begin his run. Your thought that people think you're unfriendly is also a story. There are an infinite number of stories that can be created around the facts of what actually occurred in the park.

In the scenario with the phone call to your mother, the factual elements are that you told your mother that you and your spouse have decided to have another child. There was a pause, your mother said she needed to go, and she hung up. The story is that she hung up because of what you said about having another child. Perhaps her pause and need to end the conversation had nothing to do with what you said. The story is that she was upset and did not approve of your decision. You then got angry at her because of the story you created.

Perhaps your mother ended the conversation because someone was at the door, or because she suddenly felt lightheaded and was afraid she might faint. Maybe something happened in another room that she needed to tend to immediately. Perhaps something in the oven was burning. It could be that she was so excited about the information that she wanted to cry in private. Again, there are multiple stories that could be created around the same phenomena. We choose which stories we make up, and the stories we choose have an impact on our wellness.

You're at work on a Friday and you say hi to Joe as he walks by. Joe doesn't acknowledge you, looks straight ahead, and keeps walking down the hallway. You tell another colleague what happened and say that Joe is rude for ignoring you and must be mad at you about something. All day long you think about this encounter and what you're going to say to Joe the next time you see him. Should you give him a piece of your mind? Or maybe you should just walk by him and totally ignore him. You don't see Joe for the rest of the day. That night you relate the incident to your spouse and tell him/her what a jerk Joe is.

Over the weekend you get madder and madder at Joe and keep running through your head various scenarios about what you're going to say to him on Monday and what his likely response will be. At night you have trouble falling asleep because you keep thinking about the incident on Friday and it really angers you.

Monday morning finally arrives, and as you're walking into work Joe sees you, approaches you with a big smile, and asks you how your weekend was. You ask him why he ignored you on Friday. Joe apologizes and tells you he didn't hear you speak to him, probably because he had just received a call from his wife that his son was running a fever and he was thinking about what work he needed to complete so he could go home early.

The phenomena were you said hi to Joe and he walked past you without looking at you or saying anything. The story that you created impacted your wellness on Friday and over the weekend. In addition, you may have spread your upset to your spouse, family members, and colleagues. You may also have damaged Joe's image in their eyes. You could have created a different story about the event or created no story at all.

The stories we create are important because they impact our wellness and that of those with whom we interact. We need to be able to make the distinction between phenomena and story so we can recognize when we are in a story—a fabrication around the actual facts. If we recognize that we are creating a story, we have the opportunity to choose what story we want to create. We may then decide to create a different story that serves a better purpose.

This is not to say that stories are bad and shouldn't be created. The key is to recognize when we are creating a story. If our observer is present and we see that we are creating a story, we have a choice about what story we are going to create and we have an opportunity to shift our thinking.

An option is to "create a story big enough to live in."[1] This means a story that serves both us and others in a constructive way and opens up the possibility for movement in the situation rather than a story that is restricting and that limits opportunities for positive outcomes.

Think of two situations that occurred in your life within the last few days and determine which aspects were phenomena and which were stories about the phenomena. What other stories could you have created using the same objective data that would have been more productive?

In addition to stories about specific situations, we all have stories about ourselves, about others, and about our relationships with others that we have been telling ourselves for years. We are good at locking a story into our mind and sticking with it. It may not be accurate or correct, but we believe it to be the facts and nothing but the facts. However, if we recognize that it's a story it opens up the possibility of reexamining it and creating a different story, or no story at all.

For example, a man may have an often-repeated story about himself that he is not as smart or insightful as others. As a result of that story he holds back from offering advice to others, defers to others' opinions, doesn't speak up and offer suggestions at work, and doesn't want to get a promotion and the increased responsibility. The story is limiting his behavior and life. If his story was instead that he is just as smart and insightful as others, his behavior would likely change.

Another example is a woman with a story that her spouse always purposely disagrees with her on financial decisions involving their family, so it's a waste of time to bother discussing options with him. The story may or may not be accurate. Regardless, it has limited the possibilities for their interaction and for their relationship. If a different story were created that was big enough to live in, it would open up the possibility for different actions and a change in her relationship with her husband.

What stories do you have about yourself that you've been telling yourself for years? What stories do you tell yourself about family members? About your coworkers? You have the power to create new stories that can result in a positive change in your life.

Having your observer present and being aware of the distinction between phenomena and stories empowers you to make a shift in your thinking and actions through choice. If you are aware that you're creating a story, you have the opportunity to create a more productive story.

SMALL MIND, LARGE MIND

Life throws situations and events at you all the time. You can't control their occurrence. You can, however, choose how you respond or relate to them and what actions you take in response. The choice you make has an impact on your health and wellness and the wellness of others. It also influences how others will respond or relate to you.

The following concept has power to change your thinking.

> There are at least two ways to relate to anything
> A small-minded way
> And a large-minded way
> Choose large mind[2]

As an analogy, imagine looking through a camera lens that has a knob or button which allows you to zoom in very tight on an object or pan out to a wide-angle view. You are looking at a landscape scene. You zoom in as far as you can and focus on a single blade of grass. This represents the small-minded approach. It is a very narrow and limited view of a large vista of interrelated phenomena. Now you pan out to a wide-angle view and can see the full landscape, with all the trees and flowers and grass and clouds. This represents a large-minded approach. It is a broader, more expansive view.

A small-minded way of relating to a situation is a narrow, confining, and limiting view that tends to be self-centered. A small-minded approach could be considered a downward, inward, or constricting way of looking at an event or circumstance. Small mind tends to be about me and how this situation affects me or makes me feel. It tends to be reactionary and focused on immediate gratification. A small-minded response may be your first instinct in reacting to a situation.

Choosing a small-minded view increases the likelihood of your getting a negative reaction from the other parties involved. Small mind is not open to other ways of looking at a situation and tends not to consider others or the impact on a relationship. It does not care about the consequences of your actions. It doesn't consider the possibility of a win/win outcome. It doesn't encompass the broader picture that might reveal why the situation occurred and how it evolved. It sees and reacts to the last action or event.

A large-minded way of relating to a situation is expansive and open and considers the larger picture. It tends to focus on how your actions will impact others and increases the potential for a positive outcome for all involved.

Large mind isn't reactionary. It reflects a more thought-out response that takes place after you've had a chance to digest the relevant information. It considers the reasons the event occurred and weighs the various options for how to relate to it: what actions are appropriate to effect a positive outcome. Large mind doesn't focus on what will make you feel good right now. It's about future possibilities and potential. It considers the options that will best serve.

The following exercise will demonstrate an embodied awareness of the difference between small mind and large mind.

Stand with your hands together and your clasped hands held in front of your face. Keeping your hands together, pull them downward quickly into your chest. This represents a small-minded way of relating to a situation. The movement is quick, downward, narrow, restricting, limiting, constraining, confining, and tight. It is closed and inward rather than opening into the world. It shuts down possibilities and potential for outward movement. Observe how your body feels in response to this small-minded body posture.

Now let your arms hang at your side. Shake your arms and hands and roll your shoulders to release any tension. Return to the starting position by clasping your hands and holding them in front of your face.

Now unclasp your hands and gradually raise your hands and arms over your head and outward so your body is approximating the letter Y. This posture represents a large-minded way of relating to a situation. The movement is gradual, outward, upward, broadening, widening and loose. It opens out to the world rather than closing inward. It conveys a feeling of endless possibilities and potential. Observe how different your body feels in comparison to how it felt with the small-minded movement.

Don't just imagine doing this exercise. Actually stand up and perform it. Put your body in motion. It will help you remember and embody small-minded and large-minded approaches to the situations and events of your life and demonstrate the huge difference in how your body feels. The feeling you get from assuming the small mind posture represents the impact a small-minded approach has on a situation, on others, on a relationship. Conversely, the feeling you get from the large mind movement represents the impact a large-minded approach can have. Which feeling is more comfortable? Which would appear to offer more possibilities for a positive impact on your life?

Suffering is part of life, and much of it is unavoidable: people and pets die, accidents occur, storms happen, relationships end. Life is about movement and there are events that happen that are sad and unfortunate and result in suffering. However, there is unnecessary suffering that we inflict on ourselves and on others that can be reduced. With a small-minded approach we increase unnecessary suffering; with a large-minded approach we reduce it.

Consider the situations described below in terms of a small-minded approach and a possible large-minded approach.

- You sleep through your alarm in the morning. In small mind you might run around the house yelling at everyone to hurry up.

In large mind you could tell yourself that you must have been overly tired and needed the extra sleep, then put your energy into getting everyone out on time without creating unnecessary upset.

- Your kids won't eat their breakfast. A small-minded response might be to yell at and lecture them until they leave for school. In large mind you would be aware that yelling at them may have a negative impact on their day if they go off to school upset.

- A colleague continuously complains about your boss. In small mind you may join in and adopt his habit. In large mind you could direct your conversations with him toward more positive topics and perhaps suggest actions that might result in positive changes in your boss.

- Your mother calls to complain about something insignificant. In small mind you might think she's being a real pain and is wasting your time and tell her to stop complaining. In large mind you could choose to be thankful that she's alive and has the kind of relationship with you that she calls and shares things of concern with you. You could tell her that you're interested and want to hear more so you'll call her back after work.

- At a meeting with your son's teacher she tells you that he's not very smart. A small-minded reaction might be to get aggressive, perhaps call her an idiot, and question her ability as a teacher. You might even threaten her. In large mind you might ask questions about how she came to this conclusion since you know your child is in fact very smart. You could consider what might be done to change her opinion of your child.

- Someone cuts you off and nearly causes an accident. A small-minded reaction would be to curse and follow the car, constantly honking your horn at the driver for the next fifteen minutes. You might drag your reactivity home and be angry and mad and distracted all night. In large mind you might choose to be grateful an accident didn't occur and drop the incident from your mind.

- You get to work on time for a meeting but a colleague is late because he's caught in a traffic jam. In small mind you might seize the opportunity to point out to your colleagues that you are always on time, suggesting that your coworker really messed up by being late for an important meeting. A large-minded response might be to feel sympathy for your colleague and refrain from criticizing him to your own advantage.

- Your brother calls and complains to you that his children won't sit and do their homework. In small mind you might tell him he must be doing something wrong in raising his children because your children sit and do their homework every night. In large mind you might listen sympathetically to see if you could offer helpful advice.

- You're busy doing things around the house and your children want you to come and sing to them before they go to bed. In small mind you could stay focused on everything you need to do that evening and tell your children you don't have time to sing to them. In large mind you might recognize their request as an opportunity to spend some quality time with them and acknowledge that the time you spend singing to them is more important than being able to check off all the planned activities on your to-do list.

Think of situations in which someone related to you in a small-minded fashion. What was your reaction? How did it make you feel? How did it impact the problem situation? How did it affect your relationship with them? How might they have acted in a large-minded way that would have gotten a more positive response from you?

There are many situations throughout your day when you are already choosing a large-minded approach You may be doing this instinctively without even noticing it or thinking about it. It may be natural. You may think of it as being courteous or understanding or polite or just common-sense behavior.

However, there may be situations when you tend to act in a small-minded manner. You can practice choosing large mind in these situations. Tomorrow make it your goal when you're faced with something—an event or person—that would normally induce a small-minded response to consciously choose large mind. This will require having your observer present so you recognize the opportunity to make a different choice. Choose a large-minded approach and notice how the other person reacts. Notice how you feel and how your body feels. Do the same exercise the next day. Look for opportunities to apply this practice in situations at home or at work involving family, friends or strangers.

Having our observer present helps us recognize that there is more than one possible story and more than one way of relating to a situation. We realize we have a choice and are empowered to shift to a large-minded view of the situation and its possibilities.

> There are at least two ways to relate to anything
> A small-minded way
> And a large-minded way
> Choose large mind

UPSET IS OPTIONAL

Here is an enlightening saying that may serve to create new possibilities in your life: "Upset is optional."[3] All of us get upset at some time.

All day long we encounter situations we can get upset about. In fact, we may think that we have no choice but to be upset about them. However, in reality we are choosing to be upset. No one can force us to be upset. It is a choice we make. We cannot avoid bad things and sad occurrences in our life, but we can choose how we relate to them.

To say that upset is optional is not to say that you should not choose to be upset. You may feel it serves you or the situation to be upset. However, there is a difference between being in reactionary upset which treats upset as the only option and making a conscious choice to be upset because you believe it may serve.

Involuntarily choosing to be upset has an impact on your own wellness and well-being and on that of others. When you're upset, observe the physical phenomena in your body. How does your body react? Perhaps your breathing changes. There may be a tightness or pain in your shoulders or neck. Maybe your stomach feels heavy or your face gets flushed. Perhaps you clench your teeth. Possibly your head starts to hurt. Being upset has a physical impact on your body.

Choosing not to be upset or not to stay in upset will also have an impact on your body. Observe what happens after you decide to no longer be in upset. How does your body react?

Your upset may have an impact on your relationship with others: at home, at work, with strangers. Think of a situation when someone was upset with you and how you reacted. How could they have approached the situation differently and gotten a different reaction from you? How would an alternative approach have affected your relationship? How did your body react when they were upset with you? Their upset impacted your body and therefore your health and wellness.

"Upset is optional" does not mean you ignore a situation. It means there may be other ways to relate to it. Some of the tools this book offers may help you to have a different response. You can have your observer present and choose to relate to the situation in a large-minded way. You can reframe the situation to not be upset or to reduce the amount of time you are in upset mode. The idea that upset is optional is not about making a value judgment, it is pointing to the fact that you have a choice as to whether to be upset, how upset to be, how long to be upset, and how to respond or relate to the situation. These are choices within your control.

A quote from Aristotle points to this concept. "Anyone can become angry—that is easy. But to be angry with the right person, to the right degree, at the right time, for the right purpose and in the right way— this is not easy."

Another concept that may be helpful in dealing with certain situations is, "Bow to what is." The idea is to accept and acknowledge things as they are without a judgment or emotional reaction. A popular phrase in Western culture conveying a similar message is, "It is what it is."

Expectations are a large contributor of upset in people. We may have certain expectations about a situation, a person, how things should happen, or what should occur. When the actual event is different from our expectation, we get upset. If we did not have a fixed expectation to measure the event or occurrence against, we might not be upset. Recognizing that we have created a story and expectations related to the situation provides us with a framework and opportunity to choose not to be upset.

- A friend said he would call you and he didn't. You have many options regarding how you choose to relate to this event. You can choose to be upset or you can choose to not be upset. You can choose to be furious at your friend or choose to be just a little mad. You can choose to be worried that something bad happened that kept him from calling. You can choose to be sad. You can choose to not care.

- Your child brings home a C in science on his report card. You have many options in how you choose to relate to this event. You can be very upset and scream at him. You can tell him he's not smart and send him to his room. You can tell him you expected an A and you're furious because he didn't get it. Or you can tell him that you're not mad and promise to get him some help with the work next quarter. You can tell him you know he has the potential to do better and you will work on this together. The choice you make affects your well-being and that of your son Think about the likely reaction in your body when you were a child if someone had said to you some of the things in the possible responses above. Think about the likely reaction in your son and his body.

- A coworker goes to lunch with some other colleagues and doesn't invite you. Again, you have many options. You can choose to be extremely mad that you weren't included. You can find out where they went for lunch, follow them, and scream at your coworker. You can decide not to talk to her for the rest of the day. You can leave a long letter on her desk highlighting all the rude things she has done. You can send her an e-mail telling her she has deeply hurt you. Or you can wonder why you weren't invited and ask her about it later in the day. You can tell yourself that she must have had a good reason for not inviting you and hope she's having a good time. You can decide if it serves to be upset and how you want to relate to this situation and what action you're going to take.

- You're in line at the nine-items-or-less express checkout line at the grocery store. The person in front of you starts putting his groceries on the belt and you notice that he has eighteen items. You can choose to be upset and start yelling at him to take his groceries to another checkout line. You can call for a manager. You can yell to the cashier and demand that she not ring up more than nine of his items. You can point out to the person behind you that the man in front of you is being very inconsiderate by being in the express line. Or you can say and do nothing. Whatever choice you make will impact your well-being and the well-being of the people around you.

• You live in a three-bedroom house with a small backyard. You had an expectation that at this stage of your life you would have a bigger house with a huge backyard. You have many options in relating to the discrepancy between your expectations and reality. You can be upset that you don't live in a bigger house. You can hate your house and be disappointed with this aspect of your life. You can be angry at your various employers over the years and blame them for the fact that you don't have a bigger house. You can be angry at your spouse for not making more money. You can be upset with your children and blame them for your not being able to afford a bigger house. Or you can choose to be happy that you were able to afford to buy a house. You can be happy that you haven't lost your job and can make the mortgage payments. You can consider yourself more fortunate than many people who do not have a house or one as nice as yours.

In any situation in which we find ourselves, we are empowered to choose whether or not to be upset. The choice we make impacts our health, wellness and well-being and the well-being of our family members and others. Upset is most definitely optional.

YES, YES, NOW

We all have the ability to make a change in how we relate to something, someone, some situation, or some incident. We are very practiced at locking ourselves into a story or a way of relating to something. *And* we have the power to change how we relate. It is not always easy, it is not always what we want to do, it is not always a permanent change, but each of us does in fact have the power and ability to change. It is a matter of choice.

We all have "squawks." A squawk is something that irritates you or bothers you or makes you angry. It could be a gripe, a complaint, an annoyance, an issue that results in a negative reaction in you and your body. It can be something small, such as, "It bugs me when my spouse sits and watches television all evening," or "It irritates me when my co-worker takes the last cup of coffee and doesn't start a new pot," or "It makes me mad when my child doesn't hug me back when I hug her." Or it can be something major, such as, "I'm mad at my mother for the way she's treated my spouse over the years," or "I'm infuriated with my boss for not giving me the promotion," or "I get so mad at my son every time he chooses to be with his girlfriend instead of hanging out at home with me."

We all have lots of squawks in varying degrees of importance and strength. We like to hang onto our squawks. We have perfected our story around the squawk. We are good at telling that story and we do not want to give it up.

We have a choice whether to hold onto the squawk and the story and the impact it is having on our relationships and our wellness. We can also choose to make a change and give up the squawk. No one is making us keep the squawk. It is our choice.

If you choose to make a change, here is an exercise[4] you can do either with someone else or by yourself. Making a change may require starting with baby steps, and this exercise helps take those first few steps. The exercise as described is for two people

Ask a friend to think of a particular squawk she has about someone. Have her acknowledge when she has a squawk in mind, but do not have her tell you what her squawk is. If she tells you, you will likely want to try to help her resolve the issue she has or offer advice. It's best not to know the squawk. Observe your friend's body before she thinks of the squawk. Then, after she has thought of it, note what changes you observe.

Once she has a squawk in mind, ask her, "Could you give up the squawk?" She may answer "No." In response to her "No" you ask again, "Is it possible to give up the squawk?" It *is* possible, because no one is making us hold onto a squawk. There isn't a gun being held to our head that will be fired if we give it up. It is our choice to hang on.

If she still says "No" you try again by asking, "If you wanted to, could you give up the squawk?" You aren't asking if she will actually give it up, you're just asking whether it's physically possible. In the universe we live in, is it possible that she could give up the squawk if she chose to? You want to get to the point that she says "Yes" to the question, "Could you give up the squawk?"

This is very important because once a person acknowledges and sees that it is possible to give up the squawk, it opens up tremendous possibilities. It then becomes a choice that can be made. It unlocks the concept that we are not forced to think or react or act in a certain way. We may not want to change, but if we acknowledge that a change is indeed possible, it creates the potential for a change.

The next question you ask your friend is, "Would you give up your squawk?" Typically a person will say "No," because they have lived with their squawk for a long time and don't want to get rid of it. Here is when you go after baby steps. You ask questions until you get the person to answer "Yes" to one of them. "Would you give up your squawk for one day?" "Would you give it up until you get home?" "Would you give it up for one hour?" "Would you give it up for ten minutes?"

Another way to get a yes answer is to ask your friend to think of someone who would benefit if she gave up her squawk. Perhaps it's a child, a spouse, a grandchild, a parent, a sibling, a coworker. "For the sake of this person would you give up your squawk?" This is very powerful because we will do things for the sake of those we love and care about even if we won't do them for ourselves.

"For the sake of this person would you give up your squawk for a day?" "For the sake of this person would you let go of your squawk for one hour?" "For the sake of this person would you let go of your squawk for ten minutes?" "For the sake of this person would you let go of it for one minute?" You keep crunching it down until you get a yes answer.

We all have the ability to let go of our squawk if we choose to. Choosing to let go for the sake of someone else for a short period of time is a dramatic occurrence. If we let it go for any period of time, then we have achieved movement toward letting it go for a longer period of time. This can have a positive impact on our well-being and the well-being of others.

Once you have gotten a "Yes" to the questions involving "Could you let go of your squawk?" and "Would you let go?" there is one more question you need to address. Ask your friend, "When will you give up your squawk?" She may say "Tomorrow" or "Later tonight" or attach some conditions to the person she has the squawk about. The answer you want is, "Now." If she will not give up her squawk now, then you crunch down the time frame or add names from the "for the sake of" list until she is willing to let go of her squawk right now, even if it's only for thirty seconds. Getting a "now" answer to the last question is important because she will take the action while it is fresh in her mind. If the action of letting go of her squawk is promised to be taken later, it may never happen.

After your friend agrees to let go of her squawk right now, instruct her to let it go. Watch her body. What changes do you observe in her between holding onto the squawk and letting it go?

This exercise is called "Yes, Yes, Now" because those are the answers you need to elicit to create movement toward change. Remember that you didn't know what your friend was thinking about. You aren't trying to validate or agree or disagree with the squawk or explain why it occurs. You are not trying to fix the problem.

You are helping your friend recognize that she has a choice concerning this squawk and that there may be a positive impact on her, the person who is the object of the squawk, someone else, or a relationship if she lets go of it. You are also helping her realize that it is possible to give up the squawk for at least a short period of time and the world will not come to an end. You are helping her realize that she has the power and ability to choose.

After you have gone through this exercise asking your friend to think of a squawk, switch roles. You think of a squawk and have her ask you the questions. You go through the same exercise.

You can also do this exercise by yourself. Think of a squawk and ask yourself the same questions you would ask your friend. "Could I let go of it?" "Would I let go of it for the sake of someone else?" "Will I let go of it for the sake of someone else even for a specified short period beginning right now?" Then let go of it for the designated time. You can repeat this exercise at a later time with the same squawk to see if you will let go of it for a longer period of time. You can repeat it with other squawks.

ADDRESSING STRESS

Although stress is a prevalent topic in modern society, as a health-related and medical term it has only been around since 1936.[5] A scientist named Hans Selye studied laboratory animals and noticed similarities in physical reactions of various animals to outside influences. He coined the term "stress" to mean the nonspecific response of the body to any demand for change, such as from outside forces. His research pointed to the fact that the body will automatically respond to forces in a certain way and there is consistency in this response. He did not intend stress to have a negative connotation or only apply to an unpleasant threat.

The term "stress" has been used in physics for centuries and refers to elasticity, which is the property of a material that allows it to resume its original size and shape after having been compressed or stretched. Selye, who was Hungarian born, spoke several languages, including English, but was not aware of the use of the term "stress" in physics. He admitted later in life that if he'd had a better knowledge of English he would have used the word "strain." If so, perhaps today your friend would be telling you she is "strained out."

The automatic physical response in our body to forces that Selye noted is a quality that each of us has inherited from primitive humans. We not only inherit unique characteristics and qualities from our parents, we inherit from the earliest humans ingrained and automatic reactions in our body over which we have no control. These reactions were intended to be beneficial.

When primitive humans faced danger, it was a life-threatening situation and there was an automatic and immediate physiological change in their body that enabled them to deal with imminent danger. This is what we know as the "fight or flight" response. This physiological mechanism is still intact in us.

When a person experiences a threat or danger, the brain responds and hormones are released into our system to prepare for fight or flight. The heart rate and blood pressure surge dramatically to increase the flow of blood to the brain to improve decision making. Blood is moved away from the stomach area, where it is not immediately needed for purposes of digestion, to the muscles of the arms and legs to provide more strength.

Clotting occurs more quickly to prevent blood loss from injuries. Blood sugar rises to furnish more fuel for energy. The breathing rate increases. Digestion shuts down, regenerative processes are put on hold, and reproductive urges and capabilities dwindle because they are not needed to deal with the immediate threat. The immune system is weakened. These automatic physiological changes are designed to respond to an immediate physical threat from an outside force, not to deal with long-term situations.

Our body responds similarly to psychological stress, which may be chronic rather than short-term. For example, when we sit and worry about something we turn on the same physiological responses as would occur in the presence of physical danger. These prolonged responses have a negative effect on long-term health and wellness since their function is not to maintain a healthy body but to address an immediate danger.

The ability of stress to impact health is not surprising when you consider the physiological response of the body, which, as we've noted, is designed to allow a quick response to a short-term situation and not intended to persist for a long period of time. The normal bodily functions designed to promote and sustain long-term health and growth are put on hold during this response to an immediate threat. If the body is responding to a chronic or extended psychological condition, these functions are mitigated or have a reduced impact, increasing the body's susceptibility to disease. One theory is that stress doesn't cause the disease but that the body loses its resistance to fight it.

We all experience some degree of stress in response to the pressures of life and the external and internal forces that affect us. The key questions are how to address them and what we can learn from them.

The first thing we can do is prepare our mind and body, which are interdependent, to deal with the forces we encounter that normally induce a stress response. We can create an environment in our mind and body that enables us to deal with these forces in a manner which eliminates or reduces their negative impact. We can do this through participating in regular movement and exercise, using breathing techniques, increasing the amount of sleep and rest we get, engaging meditation and relaxation practices, developing good eating and nutrition habits, and avoiding excess caffeine.

Another effective action we can take is to identify what is causing the stress and reframe how we relate to it. We may want to remove ourselves from the situation. Alternatively, we can use the techniques and practices discussed in this book to shift how we deal with it and thereby alter its impact on us. These concepts and techniques include distinguishing between phenomena and story; choosing large mind; remembering that upset is optional; bowing to what is; and practicing Yes, Yes, Now. The objective is to understand where the stress is coming from and make some kind of change to address its underlying cause rather than merely treating the symptom.

Another effective option available to us is to use our reaction to stress as a teacher. When you are experiencing stress, how does it show up in your body? Headaches? Poor sleep? Loss of interest in sex? Loss of appetite? Perhaps you lose focus or your shoulders slump. Maybe you become very emotional: weepy, irritable, or short on patience. Learn how your body responds to stress and then become acutely aware when these symptoms show up. When they appear, your body is being a teacher and sending you a very clear message that something is going on that you may want to address.

We are each empowered to take action to change how we relate to life and the impact stress will have on our health and wellness. "Stressed" spelled backwards is "desserts." Perhaps if we shift how we relate to stress, there will be a delicious, unexpected outcome.

Clearly we have many choices in how we relate to life's situations and to other people. Shifting to being aware that you have a choice and that your choice has an impact on your health and wellness and on that of those you interact with is a great first step. The next is to actually make positive life choices.

REFLECTIONS

⌇

GLASS JARS

There once was a wise teacher, whose words of wisdom students would come from far and wide to hear. One day as usual, many students began to gather in the teaching room. They came in and sat down very quietly, looking to the front with keen anticipation, ready to hear what the teacher had to say.

Eventually the teacher came in and sat down in front of the students. The room was so quiet you could hear a pin drop. On one side of the teacher was a large glass jar. On the other side was a pile of dark grey rocks. Without saying a word, the teacher began to pick up the rocks one by one and place them very carefully in the glass jar. When all the rocks were in the jar, the teacher turned to the students and asked, "Is the jar full?" "Yes, the jar is full," said the students.

Without saying a word, the teacher began to drop small round pink pebbles carefully into the large glass jar so that they fell down between the rocks. When all the pebbles were in the jar, the teacher turned to the students and asked, "Is the jar now full?" The students looked at one another and said, "Yes, teacher, the jar is now full."

Without saying a word, the teacher took some fine silver sand and let it trickle into the large glass jar where it settled around the pink pebbles and the dark grey rocks. When all the sand was in the jar, the teacher turned to the students and asked, "Is the jar now full?" A few students confidently said, "Yes, the jar is now full. Now it is definitely full."

Without saying a word, the teacher took a jug of water and poured it carefully, without splashing a drop, into the large glass jar. When the water reached the brim, the teacher turned to the students and asked, "Is the jar now full?" Most of the students were silent, but two students ventured to answer, "Yes, the jar is now finally full."

Without saying a word, the teacher took a handful of salt and sprinkled it slowly over the top of the water. When all the salt had dissolved into the water, the teacher turned to the students and asked once more, "Is the jar now full?" Eventually one brave student said, "Yes, teacher. The jar is now full."

"Yes, the jar is now full," said the teacher.

The teacher then told the students, "A story always has many meanings, and you will each have understood many things from this demonstration. Discuss amongst yourselves what meanings the story has for you. How many different messages can you find in it and take from it?"

The students looked at the wise teacher and at the beautiful glass jar filled with grey rocks, pink pebbles, silver sand, water and salt. Then they discussed with each other the meanings the story had for them. After a few minutes, the wise teacher raised one hand and the room fell silent. The teacher said, "Remember that there is never just one interpretation of anything. You have all taken away many meanings and messages from the story, and each meaning is as important and as valid as any other."[6]

Now is no time to think of what you do not have.
Think of what you can do with what there is.

~ERNEST HEMINGWAY

Holding on to anger is like holding on to a hot coal with the intent
of throwing it at someone else; you are the one who gets burned.

~BUDDHA

Reconciliation is to understand both sides: to go to one side and describe
the suffering being endured by the other side, and then go to the other
side and describe the suffering being endured by the first side.

~THICH NHAT HANH

The last of the human freedoms—to choose one's attitude in
any given set of circumstances, to choose one's own way.

~VIKTOR FRANKL

I'm an old man and I've had many troubles,
most of which never happened.

~MARK TWAIN

A pessimist is one who makes difficulties of his opportunities, and
an optimist is one who makes opportunities of his difficulties.

~HARRY TRUMAN

Anyone can become angry—that is easy. But to be angry with
the right person, to the right degree, at the right time, for the
right purpose and in the right way—this is not easy.

~ARISTOTLE

My barn having burned to the ground, I can now see the moon.

~CHINESE PROVERB

We cannot choose the things that will happen to us, but we can

choose the attitude we will take toward anything that happens.
~ALFRED MONTAPERT

Life is not a matter of having good cards, but of playing a poor hand well.
~ROBERT LOUIS STEVENSON

*It takes a real storm in the average person's life to make him
realize how much worrying he has done over the squalls.*
~UNKNOWN

*Even the most enlightened beings, even the holiest saints, make
mistakes. But whereas foolish people cover up their mistakes and
keep on making the same ones, the wise correct their mistakes
and never make the same ones twice. The ability to correct
our mistakes and to change ourselves is called wisdom.*
~UNKNOWN

*When one door of happiness closes, another opens,
but often we look so long at the closed door that we do
not see the one that has been opened for us.*
~HELEN KELLER

We are the choices we make.
~MERYL STREEP

*When the pickpocket sees the saint on the road, all
the pickpocket sees is the saint's pockets.*
~SUFI SAYING

*People deal too much with the negative, with what is wrong . . .Why not try
and see positive things, to just touch those things and make them bloom?*
~THICH NHAT HANH

What happens is not as important as how you react to what happens.
~THADDEUS GOLAS

SHIFT 5

Living

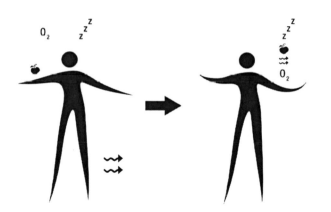

CHAPTER 5

Shift 5: LIVING

Shift: Routine daily activities impact your health and wellness.

There are routine daily activities performed by all humans that we take for granted—behaviors that have the power to impact our health and wellness. The beauty of these activities is that we do not need a medical or healthcare practitioner to prescribe them. If asked, many people would likely acknowledge that although they are generally aware that they could improve their wellness by changing their behaviors, they don't do it. The goal of this chapter is to provide you with information on why and how everyday activities and behaviors impact your health and wellness. Being informed may give you a new perspective that creates an opening for you to shift your thinking and actions.

MOVEMENT AND EXERCISE

Physical activity, exercise and movement can have a significant impact on your wellness and well-being. The World Health Organization (WHO) defines physical activity as any bodily movement produced by skeletal muscles that requires energy expenditure. They report that physical inactivity is an independent risk factor for chronic diseases, and overall is estimated to cause 1.9 million deaths globally.

According to WHO, physical activity is a key determinant of energy expenditure and thus is fundamental to energy balance and weight control. Physical activity reduces the risk of coronary heart disease, stroke, type 2 diabetes, colon cancer, and breast cancer in women. There is even evidence to suggest that increasing levels of various types of physical activity may benefit health by reducing hypertension, osteoporosis and risk of falls; improving body weight and composition; and decreasing the incidence of musculoskeletal conditions such as osteoarthritis and low back pain. Physical exercise also benefits mental and psychological health by reducing depression, anxiety and stress and by increasing control over risky behaviors (e.g., tobacco use, alcohol and other substance abuse, unhealthy diet choices).

The World Health Organization further states that regular physical activity can improve women's health and help prevent many of the diseases and conditions that are major causes of death and disability for women throughout the world. Many women suffer from disease processes that are associated with inadequate participation in physical activity such as cardiovascular disease, diabetes, and osteoporosis. Cardiovascular diseases account for one-third of deaths among women around the world and half of all deaths in women over fifty years of age in developing countries. Diabetes affects more than 70 million women worldwide, and its prevalence is projected to double by 2025. Osteoporosis is a disease in which bones become fragile and more likely to break and is most prevalent in postmenopausal women.

WHO recommends thirty minutes of moderate-intensity physical activity five days per week to improve and maintain health. The thirty minutes can be accumulated over the course of a day in blocks as short as ten minutes.[1]

We tend to think of exercise as running, playing a sport, swimming, using workout equipment, or some other activity that requires extensive physical exertion. There are other options which have a benefit, including walking, low-impact exercise, or other mild fitness practices.

In addition to the conventional forms of exercise popular in the West, there is another type of activity that promotes wellness. In China there are two movement programs that have been used for thousands of years and are becoming very popular in Western cultures: t'ai chi and qigong. Although these programs benefit everyone, they are particularly useful for people who don't like to exercise or who have problems with conventional exercises because of physical ailments. These programs impact not only the body but also the mind. An acupuncturist will frequently suggest that a patient participate in some movement program or class to promote the body's healing process.

T'ai chi (pronounced tie chee) is an ancient program of gentle, slow, fluid movements and coordinated breathing. The movements are designed to stimulate the flow of the energy force (chi or qi) and to promote balance in mind and body. T'ai chi originated as a martial arts style and has been adopted as a movement program because of its health benefits.

The opening ceremonies to the 2008 Olympic Games in Beijing, China, included 2,008 t'ai chi experts demonstrating its graceful and fluid movements. In parks in China it is common to see groups of people practicing t'ai chi in the morning.

Qigong (pronounced chee gung) is another ancient movement program based on gentle movements with coordinated breathing that includes visualization. It has been described as a self-healing art that, like t'ai chi, cultivates the energy force within us and plays an active role in maintaining health.

When gentle movements are integrated with full, relaxed breathing and deep relaxation of mind, the body enters an especially healing and restorative state. This has a positive effect on the blood, the nervous system, the immune system, and oxygen metabolism.

Yoga is another practice that may serve you. Yoga is a mind-body practice with origins in ancient Indian philosophy. The various styles of yoga that people use for health purposes typically combine physical postures, breathing techniques, and meditation or relaxation.[2]

In addition to formal movement programs, there are movements you can perform at various times during the day to promote your wellness. For example:

- At work, sit at your desk, hold a stapler in your hand and lift it over your head ten times. Then switch to the other hand.
- While sitting at your desk, stretch your legs out in front of you and lift them off the ground. Point your toes forward and then straight up.
- While sitting or standing, pat your legs with your hands, starting at your waist and moving down to your feet. Then pat your legs moving back up to your waist.
- While sitting or standing, roll your shoulders forward five times, rest, then roll them back five times.
- While sitting or standing, let your arms rest at your side and then shake them.

Incorporate additional physical activity or exercise and movement into your routine and see what you notice. How does your body react? What changes do you note in your thinking, emotions and mood? How does it affect your sleeping? What effect does it have on any symptoms you may have been experiencing? What changes does it make in how you handle stress? In how you relate to situations?

Physical activity, exercise, and movement have an impact on the conditions within your body and mind and therefore on your health and wellness. These are activities available to you that promote the natural healing of your body and do not require a medical practitioner.

BREATHING

Breathing is an activity most of us don't think about, but there are many ways to breathe and we breathe differently in different situations.

- The professional basketball player is at the free-throw line about to take a foul shot that could win the game. He goes through his standard routine. He dribbles the ball three times. He takes a deep breath. He shoots.

- The Olympic swimmer is on the starting box getting ready to dive into the pool for the race she has been training for her entire life. She shakes her legs. She swings her arms in a windmill fashion. She takes a deep breath. She gets into her starting position to be ready to dive in at the sound of the starting gun.

- The comedian is standing behind the curtain getting ready to go on stage. The announcer introduces him to the crowd and the audience claps. He takes a deep breath and steps out onto the stage.

- A teenager is on the phone with his girlfriend and she breaks up with him. He begins crying very intensely and runs downstairs to tell his mother. He is so upset he can barely speak. His mother tells him, "Breathe, breathe. Now tell me what happened."

- An adult daughter is talking to her mother, who is commenting on how the daughter is raising her children. After one particular comment that hits a nerve, the daughter thinks to herself,

"Breathe. Count to three and breathe."

- A man has just been in a car accident and is very upset and pan-icked. He is breathing very shallowly and rapidly. To get him to calm down his spouse instructs him to take long deep breaths.

These are situations that clearly reflect that we breathe differently in different situations. When we get upset or busy or panicked or nervous, our breathing tends to become shallow. When we want to relax or calm ourselves, we may take a slow deep breath.

Breathing a certain way can assist us in how we relate to a situation, and therefore impact our wellness. Changing how we are breathing can relax the body, help our mind focus, change our emotional state, and reduce the impact of stress. Changing how we are breathing can foster the self-healing powers of our body.

For thousands of years, ancient cultures emphasized special breath-ing practices because they were found to have value for a person's health and wellness.[3] Eastern meditation, relaxation, and movement practices, including yoga, t'ai chi, and qigong, incorporate breathing as an integral component of the activity.

We take over 17,000 breaths a day. In addition to providing us with oxygen, breathing triggers numerous physiological mechanisms.[4] Most of us have learned to breathe a certain way and we can learn to breathe in alternative ways. Changing the way we breathe can result in physi-ological changes that benefit us.

We take in oxygen through our mouth or nose. The process of breath-ing takes place mainly in the chest cavity, which includes the lungs, dia-phragm and rib cage. The top and sides of the chest cavity house the ribs and intercostal muscles. The bottom of the chest cavity includes the dome-shaped diaphragm. Inside the chest cavity is the heart and two lungs. The diaphragm is located in your abdomen area.

Two basic ways of breathing are chest breathing and deep breathing. Many people use shallow chest breathing.

Deep breathing is sometimes called diaphragmatic breathing, natural breathing, or abdominal breathing. The breath is focused in the diaphragm rather than in the chest. Deep breathing serves to trigger relaxation, which causes the blood capillaries to expand, allowing more oxygen to travel to locations where healing is needed. Deep breathing using our diaphragm efficiently pulls oxygen into all areas of our lungs, which is more beneficial than shallow chest breathing.[5]

Deep breathing is more effective in pumping lymph fluid throughout the body, which stimulates self-healing. The lymph fluid contains immune cells which are targeted to fight bacteria and viruses. In addition, deep breathing shifts the production of brain chemicals which promote healing.[6]

When we mainly use shallow upper-chest breathing, we reduce the efficiency of our lungs and the respiratory system. Compared to deep breathing, shallow breathing results in less blood flow and less productive distribution of the vital lymph fluids. It also reduces the amount of digestive juices available for the digestive process and weakens the functioning of various systems in the body.

Here are two ways to tell if you're a chest breather or a diaphragm breather. Place your right hand on your upper chest and your left hand on your abdomen in your navel area. Breathe normally. If the right hand rises first, you are upper-chest breathing. If the left hand rises first, you are deep diaphragm breathing. Another method is to see which hand rises more. If your right hand rises more, you're a chest breather. If your left hand rises more, you are an abdomen breather. Now perform the exercise by breathing slowly through your nose and see if you notice a difference.

To relax and practice deep breathing, take a slow deep breath through your nose and fill the lower portion of your lungs first and then fill the upper portion of your lungs. Then exhale slowly through your nose. Repeat the exercise. This practice is best performed lying on your back or sitting erect.

Another breathing exercise is to lie on your back and, as in the previous exercise, take a slow deep breath through your nose and fill the lower portion of your lungs first, then the upper portion. Exhale through your mouth instead of through your nose, making a sound as you empty the air out of your lungs. Repeat the exercise.

You can use deep breathing to create an environment in your body favorable to healing. You can use it to reduce the impact of stress, relax and calm yourself, stop an automatic reaction to a situation and create a pause to allow you to act rather than react, stop a negative thought from occurring or minimize its effect, and refocus your mind.

During the day take deep breaths and see how your body and mind respond.

SLEEP AND REST

Although getting adequate sleep and rest is essential to health and wellness, most people take it for granted. Some consider it a waste of time. Your body has remarkable healing power, and rest and sleep play a large part in the healing process. When you don't get enough, it impacts your body's healthy functioning.

You no doubt have engaged in conversations with people about the effects of sleep deprivation. You're talking to a friend and notice he's a bit irritable. You ask him if he's annoyed with you and he says, "Nothing's wrong, I just haven't gotten much sleep the last few nights." A colleague leaves work early and tells you on the way out, "I'm dragging and could use a good night's sleep." Your spouse apologizes for being short-tempered and snapping at you, and you respond, "Nothing a good night's sleep won't fix." A workaholic neighbor goes at a nonstop pace for weeks, takes a weekend off, and tells you, "I just needed to re-charge my battery."

The National Sleep Foundation maintains that seven to nine hours of sleep per night is optimal for most adults and that sufficient sleep promotes overall health and alertness. The brain has an internal bio-logical clock which regulates the timing of our sleep. It impacts body temperature and enzyme distribution and determines the ideal time for restorative sleep.[7] The body prefers to follow the natural cycles of day and night, so seven hours of sleep between the hours of 11 pm and 6 am is more productive and efficient than seven hours of sleep between 2 am and 9 am.[8]

Sleep debt is the result of not getting enough rest and sleep and can cause physical, emotional and mental fatigue. Studies have shown that sleep loss impairs immune function and the healing process.

When we sleep, our blood pressure is lowered, hormones are se-creted, kidney functions change, sensory and motor activity are rela-tively suspended, and the immune system is impacted. The hormones produced during sleep promote growth, help build muscle mass, repair cells and tissues, and work to fight infections.[9] Sufficient sleep not only promotes healing when you are ill or sick but helps create a positive en-vironment in your body which may reduce the occurrence or severity of disease or illness.

If you think about it, you see signs of the importance of sleep on the body's ability to function throughout life. Babies sleep a lot because sleep is important for their growth and development. Teenagers tend to need more sleep than adults during their growing years. When you have a cold or aren't feeling well, you intuitively sense that you need extra sleep to help you recover.

All bodies are unique in how much sleep they need to function optimally. Your body knows how much sleep you need and will be your teacher and alert you when you aren't getting enough. What shows up in your body when you have had insufficient sleep? What happens to the symptoms you experience and how does your body respond after you get more sleep? What is the effect on your mind and thinking when you're sleep deprived? How does lack of sleep impact your attitude and temperament?

Many of us are instinctively aware of the need for more sleep but choose to ignore it. If you don't respond to early messages from your body, more serious problems could develop.

Don't underestimate the impact of sleep on your health, wellness, and well-being. Sleep is a treatment you can provide to yourself. It doesn't cost anything, doesn't require a prescription, doesn't require instructions from a doctor, and is available to everyone.

FOOD AND WELLNESS

Food can have a dramatic effect on our health, wellness, and well-being. What we eat and drink affects our mood, our reaction to stress, our sleep, and our risk of disease.

Most of us are aware that what we eat or drink has an effect on our body, even if we don't think of it in terms of our health and wellness. How does your body respond to an extremely spicy meal? To a huge steak? To a hot bowl of soup when you have a cold? To drinking alcohol? To consuming coffee? To eating a large meal shortly before going to bed? What is its response to skipping meals? What happens to your mood when you skip meals? When you eat too many items high in sugar?

Common sense and research lead us to conclude that what we eat and drink has an impact on the systems and conditions of our body. Therefore, it clearly has an impact on our health and wellness.

Chronic diseases are linked to the "Western diet." A Western diet is generally defined as a diet consisting of an abundance of processed food, red meat, refined grains, fat and sugar, and plenty of everything except vegetables, fruits and whole grains. Populations that eat a Western diet suffer from higher rates of cardiovascular disease, cancer, type 2 diabetes, and obesity than people eating traditional diets within a wide range of cultures.[10]

The World Health Organization reports that diet is second only to tobacco as a preventable cause of cancer. They note that diets high in fruit and vegetables may reduce the risk for various types of cancer, while high levels of preserved and/or red meat consumption are associated with increased cancer risk.[11]

There are many books, articles, magazines, and websites focused on the effect of diet on our health and wellness. There are enormous amounts of research demonstrating the impact of nutrition on various aspects of our health and life. While there may be differences of opinion as to what constitutes a proper diet or what the specific impact of any particular food is, there is general agreement that what we eat and drink does in fact matter and will have an impact on our health.

Many experts agree that health is promoted by eating more vegetables and fruits, chemical-free food, more whole foods, and less processed food. There are studies demonstrating that a diet rich in vegetables and fruits reduces the risk of dying from diseases common in the West. For example, in countries in which people eat a pound or more of vegetables and fruit a day, the rate of cancer is half of what it is in the United States.[12] In addition, an estimated 80 percent of cases of type 2 diabetes could be prevented by a change in diet and exercise.[13]

Whole foods are those in the form that nature provides, with all their edible parts. Whole foods of vegetable origin include fresh vegetables and fruits; whole grains (millet, brown rice, oats, rye, whole wheat, buckwheat, quinoa, cornmeal); beans and legumes (lentils, chick peas, kidney and other beans); nuts and seeds. Whole foods of animal origin include eggs, small whole fish, seafood (shrimp, lobster, soft shell crabs), and small fowl.

According to some experts, eating whole foods promotes getting the largest amount of nutrients in their natural form in the right proportions.[14] Conversely, fragmented foods include all foods that are missing original parts, as in refined carbohydrates such as white flour and white rice, which are missing the fiber and nutrients found in the bran and germ.[15]

The importance of food on health and wellness has been recognized in cultures throughout recorded history. Hippocrates acknowledged the role of food when he said, "Let your food be your medicine and let your medicine be your food."

In China, food has been used for centuries not only for nourishment but also for healing and wellness. An ancient Chinese medical text reflects the importance of food on health and wellness, stating, "If people pay attention to the five flavors and mix them well, their bones will remain straight, their muscles will remain tender and young, their breath will circulate freely, their pores will be fine in texture, and consequently, their breath and bones will be filled with the essence of life."[16]

The key point is that what we eat does in fact have an impact on our health and wellness and we should not take lightly the choices we make. This is an area in which we are all empowered to have a positive effect on our own wellness by making changes that promote our health without the aid of a medical practitioner. A meal is not just food; it is a vital ingredient in your health and wellness.

There are numerous resources available on the subject of food and nutrition. For your own sake and that of your family, you can become an educated "*consumer.*"

The routine daily activities of moving, breathing, sleeping, and eating affect our health and wellness. Making a shift to recognize their potential and to make appropriate changes in these areas will have a positive impact.

REFLECTIONS

THE STREAM

Two Zen monks were returning to their monastery after a long journey. As they came upon a swift running stream, a lovely young woman came toward them from a grove of trees where she had been waiting. "Noble sirs," she said, "I am traveling to aid my mother who has fallen ill. She lives across the stream and to the south. But the stream is so swollen that I cannot cross for fear I shall be swept away. Will you help me cross, good sirs?"

The elder of the two monks nodded graciously, picked up the young woman and carried her across the raging stream. On the other side, he lowered her gently to the ground. The young woman expressed her thanks and continued on her way toward the south.

The two monks wished her well and turned to the north to continue their journey home. Neither spoke for a few hours. The younger monk was sullen and silent as they walked along. After hours had passed, the younger of the two scolded his companion, "You are aware that we monks do not touch women. Why did you carry that girl?" The elder monk smiled and said, "I lifted her up and put her down hours ago. Why are you still carrying her?"[17]

IT TAKES A VILLAGE

In a tribe in South Africa, when a person acts irresponsibly or un-justly, he is placed in the center of the village. All work stops and every man, woman and child in the village gathers in a large circle around the accused individual. Then each person in the tribe speaks to the ac-cused, one at a time, about all the good things the person in the center has done in his lifetime. Every experience and every incident that can be recalled is told. All his positive attributes, good deeds, strengths and kindnesses are recited carefully and at length. The ceremony often lasts several days. At the end, the tribal circle is broken, a joyous celebration takes place, and the person is symbolically and literally welcomed back into the tribe.[18]

❧

Live each season as it passes: breathe the air, drink the drink,
taste the fruit, and resign yourself to the influences of each.
~HENRY DAVID THOREAU

The ability to be in the present moment is a
major component of mental wellness.
~ABRAHAM MASLOW

The doctor of the future will give no medicine but will
interest his patient in the care of the human frame, in
diet, and in the cause and prevention of disease.
~GEORGE BERNARD SHAW

Dream no small dreams for they have no power to move the hearts of men.
~JOHANN WOLFGANG VON GOETHE

Tell me, and I'll forget. Show me, and I may not

remember. *Involve me, and I'll understand.*
~NATIVE AMERICAN PROVERB

Activity and sadness are incompatible.
~CHRISTIAN BOVEE

In modern life, people think that their body belongs to them and they can do anything they want to it. When they make such a determination, the law supports them . . . But . . . your body is not yours alone. It also belongs to your ancestors, your parents, future generations, and all other living beings . . . Keeping your body healthy is the best way to express your gratitude to the generations.
~THICH NHAT HANH

Life moves pretty fast; if you don't stop and look around every once in a while, you could miss it.
~JOHN HUGHES

A human being is part of a whole, the "universe." Our task must be to free ourselves from the delusion of separateness to embrace all living creatures and the whole of nature.
~ALBERT EINSTEIN

Breathe. Let go. And remind yourself that this very moment is the only one you know you have for sure.
~OPRAH WINFREY

SHIFT 6

Possibilities

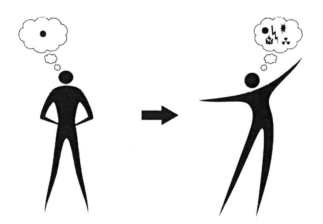

CHAPTER 6

Shift 6: POSSIBILITIES

Shift: Wellness modalities come in many forms.

Throughout the world and throughout time there have existed many healing and wellness practices and modalities. As part of being empowered to control your own health and wellness and becoming an active participant in that pursuit, it is useful to be aware of modalities that are not considered part of traditional Western medical practice. The intention of this chapter is to provide you with a brief introduction to additional modalities so you are aware they exist and can do further research on those that are of interest to you. In addition to the general overview, two specific areas—acupuncture and herbs—are covered in more detail. Shifting to a wider view of the range of wellness modalities available may serve to create additional possibilities in considering what actions you might take to enhance your health and wellness.

WELLNESS MODALITIES

There are many healing and wellness practices and modalities that have been used for generations throughout the world. Some people may discount their value or validity because they are not part of the Western medical model or appear less scientific than conventional biomedicine. Some may discount their potential because they don't understand how or why they work or don't know anyone who has tried them. Some feel there is not sufficient research to back them as viable alternatives.

Many of these modalities are based on a wellness model that reflects the healing power of the body. Many have survived the test of time. Some of them have a longer track record of successful results throughout the world than many Western technologies.

The emphasis on biomedicine as practiced in the United States and the current method of training medical doctors is fairly recent, dating back to 1910. In the 1800s and early part of the twentieth century various approaches to medicine and healing were practiced and accepted in the US, including homeopathy, osteopathy, naturopathy, and natural healing techniques which had been handed down and used for generations. There were schools that taught these techniques and they included women and minorities.

In 1910 a report was issued based on a study of the medical schools in the United States and Canada.[1] The report, which was authored by Abraham Flexner and became known as the Flexner Report, was issued by the Carnegie Foundation for the Advancement of Teaching based on a request from an organization created by the American Medical Association. At the time of the report, medical schools throughout North America varied in their admission policies, methods of teaching, curricula, assessment methodologies, graduation requirements, and ownership structure.

The report detailed the results obtained from a review of the medical schools and made a number of recommendations to standardize them based on only one model—a scientific model. The report also recommended that all medical schools be nonprofit and adhere to the protocols of mainstream science in their teaching and research. One of its conclusions was that there were too many medical schools and that too many doctors were being trained. State medical boards adopted and enforced the recommendations from the report.

The impact of the Flexner Report was that medical schools were required to adhere to high scientific standards. This meant that only one model of medicine and healing became acceptable. Other forms not based on the pure scientific approach were discouraged. Many of the schools that had been teaching other modalities were closed, and these disciplines were dropped from the schools that remained in operation.

As a result of the report, about 45 percent of medical schools closed within the next ten years, and 57 percent within 25 years. In the first ten years following the release of the report the number of medical doctors being trained was reduced by over 50 percent. Another impact was that the cost of attending medical school increased, and students admitted were predominantly white males. The number of women, minorities and low-income individuals enrolling in medical schools was dramatically reduced.

There is now a growing trend in Western culture to look beyond the typical Western medical model. There is a movement toward considering other modalities, disciplines and practices to impact health, wellness, and well-being. In general, these modalities are based on a wellness model that reflects the healing power of the body and the critical importance of its inner environment or conditions.

Acupuncture

Acupuncture is a 4,000-year-old wellness procedure originating in

China that is based on balancing the *chi* (energy life force) within the body. Very thin needles are inserted into various points of the body to impact the flow of chi and maintain or restore a proper balance. According to the 2007 National Health Interview Survey, an estimated 3.2 million Americans used acupuncture in the previous year.[2]

Allopathic Medicine

Allopathic medicine refers to conventional Western medicine which is based on scientific analysis and biomedicine. The term *allopathy* means "other than the disease" and was coined by the founder of homeopathy to differentiate between the philosophy of homeopathy and that of conventional medicine.

Ayurvedic Medicine

Ayurvedic medicine is a 5,000-year-old medical system founded in India which aims to integrate and balance the body, mind, and spirit. It uses a variety of products and techniques to cleanse the body and restore balance. To prevent illness, Ayurvedic medicine emphasizes hygiene, exercise, herbal preparations, and yoga. To cure ailments, it relies on herbal medicines and diet. Ayurvedic treatment goals include eliminating impurities, reducing symptoms, increasing resistance to disease, and increasing harmony in the patient's life. According to the 2007 National Health Interview Survey, more than 200,000 Americans used Ayurvedic medicine in the previous year.[3]

Chiropractic

Chiropractic is a health care approach that focuses on disorders of the musculoskeletal and nervous systems and the effects of these disorders on general health. Although practitioners may use a variety of treatment approaches, they primarily perform adjustments to the spine or other parts of the body with the goal of correcting alignment problems and supporting the body's natural ability to heal itself.[4]

Craniosacral Therapy

Craniosacral therapy is a noninvasive method of evaluating and enhancing the function of the craniosacral system. Its goal is to assist the body's natural capacity for self repair. The craniosacral system consists of the membranes and cerebrospinal fluid that surround and protect the brain and spinal cord. It extends from the bones of the skull, face, and mouth—which make up the cranium—down to the sacrum, or tailbone. The craniosacral therapy practitioner uses a light touch to assist the natural movement of fluid within the craniosacral system.[5]

Herbalism

Herbalism, used for thousands of years throughout the world, is the art and science of collecting, preparing, and utilizing herbs to promote wellness. Herbs and plants can be prepared and used in many ways. They can be taken internally as tinctures, teas, powders, syrups, or capsules.

Homeopathic Medicine

Homeopathy is a system of medical therapy that seeks to stimulate the body's ability to heal itself by giving very small doses of highly diluted substances. Homeopathic remedies are derived from natural substances that come from plants, minerals, or animals. Homeopathy is based on the principle of *similars* ("like cures like"), which states that a disease can be cured by a substance that produces similar symptoms in healthy people. According to the 2007 National Health Interview Survey, an estimated 4.8 million Americans used homeopathy in the previous year.[6]

Massage Therapy

Massage therapy is a system of structured palpation or movement of the soft tissue of the body for the benefit of the musculoskeletal, circulatory-lymphatic, nervous, and other systems of the body. Massage therapists press, rub, and otherwise manipulate the muscles and other soft tissues of the body. According to the 2007 National Health Interview Survey, an estimated 18.7 million Americans received massage therapy in the previous year.[7]

Meditation

Meditation refers to a variety of techniques or practices intended to focus or control attention. These techniques have been used by many different cultures throughout the world for thousands of years. Generally, a person who is meditating uses certain techniques, such as a specific posture, focused attention, and an open attitude toward distractions. Some forms of meditation instruct the practitioner to become mindful of thoughts, feelings, and sensations and to observe them in a nonjudgmental way.[8]

Naturopathic Medicine

Naturopathic medicine is based on the belief that the human body has an innate healing ability. Naturopathic doctors teach their patients to use diet, exercise, lifestyle changes and natural therapies to enhance the body's ability to ward off and combat disease. Naturopathic physicians base their practice on six principles: (1) Promote the healing power of nature; (2) First do no harm; (3) Treat the whole person; (4) Treat the cause; (5) Prevention is the best cure; and (6) The physician is a teacher.[9]

Oriental Medicine

Oriental medicine generally refers to the practice of combining a range of medical practices originating in China and includes the integration of acupuncture and Chinese herbs.

Osteopathic Medicine

Osteopathic medicine is a whole-person approach to health with a strong emphasis on the interrelationship of the body's nerves, muscles, bones, and organs. Doctors of osteopathic medicine believe the body's structure plays a critical role in its ability to function and are trained to identify structural problems and take action to support the body's natural tendency toward health and self-healing. They apply the philosophy of treating the whole person to the prevention, diagnosis and treatment of illness, disease and injury.[10]

Qigong

Qigong (pronounced chee gung) is a movement practice which combines gentle flowing movements, breathing, and visualization working together to create movement of chi (energy life force) to promote wellness. It has been referred to as "moving meditation."

Reflexology

Reflexology is based on an ancient Chinese therapy that involves manipulation of specific reflex areas in the foot, hands, and ears that correspond to other parts of the body. It works with the body's energy flow to stimulate self-healing and maintain balance in physical function and involves application of pressure to reflex zones to stimulate body organs and relieve areas of congestion.[11]

Reiki

Reiki (pronounced ray-key) is a Japanese technique based on the idea that there is a universal (or source) energy that supports the body's innate healing abilities. Practitioners seek to access this energy, allowing it to flow to the body and facilitate healing. They place their hands lightly on or just above the person receiving treatment with the goal of facilitating his or her own healing response. According to the 2007 National Health Interview Survey, more than 1.3 million Americans used an energy-healing therapy such as Reiki in the previous year.[12]

T'ai Chi

T'ai chi (pronounced tie chee) is an ancient Chinese movement practice that combines slow gentle movements with breathing. Practitioners move their bodies slowly, gently, and with awareness while breathing deeply in order to promote wellness. Along with qigong, it has been referred to as "moving meditation."[13]

Yoga

Yoga is a mind-body practice with origins in ancient Indian philosophy. The various styles of yoga that people use for health purposes typically combine physical postures, breathing techniques, and meditation or relaxation. The intent of yoga practices is to balance the mind, body, and spirit. According to the 2007 National Health Interview Survey, more than 14.5 million Americans used yoga in the previous year.[14]

Zero Balancing

Zero Balancing is a hands-on bodywork system designed to align the energy body with the physical structure by addressing the energy flow of the skeletal system. By working with bone energy, zero balancing seeks to correct imbalances between energy and structure, providing relief from pain, anxiety, and stress. The practitioner will gently apply pressure to various locations of the body, focusing on joints and bones.[15]

ACUPUNCTURE

Acupuncture has been successfully used in Eastern cultures for over 4,000 years. In acupuncture practice, sterile needles the diameter of a hair are gently inserted into various points of the body.

The principle behind Chinese medicine, including acupuncture, is that there is a life force called chi (pronounced chee, sometimes spelled qi or ch'i) that flows through the body, ideally in a harmonious, balanced way. The chi flows through "meridians"—which are like rivers—throughout the body. When the chi/life force is not flowing properly, there is disharmony and imbalance which impacts the body and the mind. This is illness or "dis-ease."

The theory behind acupuncture is that the body has the ability to heal itself and the acupuncture needle is helping the body get the chi in balance, which assists the healing process. There are 365 acupuncture points along the meridians that have specified names and purposes. Placing the acupuncture needles in these acupuncture points is intended to alter the flow of chi.

Acupuncture is used not only to treat diseases or ailments but to prevent them from occurring by correcting energy imbalances early. In ancient China, acupuncturists emphasized prevention and were paid to keep you well. If you were sick, they were not paid for their service during the period of your sickness.

There are common expressions in our culture that suggest an awareness of the flow of chi through the body. Someone who is having trouble writing or moving forward on a project might say, "I'm blocked." Someone who doesn't feel right but has trouble explaining it might say, "I'm out of balance." Someone who can't think of something might say, "I have a mental block," or "I'm stuck."

Although there are different approaches to acupuncture, it is essentially a holistic model which considers various aspects of the individual seeking treatment. It is based on the premise that an ailment or symptom is not occurring in a vacuum but is revealing something to the person.

The usual way in which we know that we are ill is by experiencing a symptom which acts as a signal of distress telling us that something is wrong. We may feel the distress as a migraine headache, an ulcer, a period of depression, arthritis, insomnia or some other somatic complaint. From the Eastern point of view, these symptoms point to trouble somewhere in the flow of chi.

Acupuncture is a complex system of examination, diagnosis and treatment. The acupuncturist does a full examination of the client using the diagnostic tools of Eastern medicine to assess the condition of the chi energy. This examination takes into consideration everything about the person: the sound of the voice, the hues of the face, the predominant emotion, the temperature and texture of the skin, the gait and posture, childhood history, favorite tastes, the best and worst times of day, dreams, appetite and diet, the ability to sleep, the workings of the bowel and bladder, sexual energy, stresses within the family and at work, the acuity of the senses, and habits and hobbies.[16]

The acupuncturist will typically do a comprehensive interview with the client to gather various pieces of information. The questions may include: What is your age? Do you have any other problems or complaints? What is your medical history? How would you describe yourself emotionally? What seasons do you like or not like? At what time of day do you feel better or worse? Have you noticed any changes in your eyes or sight recently? How is your skin? Do you wake up tired? Do you smoke and how often? Do you drink alcohol and how much? Do you take any medications? How is your general energy level?[17]

The answers to these and other questions may not seem relevant to you or appear to be related to the reason for your visit, but they provide valuable information to the acupuncturist. The acupuncturist will also perform pulse diagnosis.

Pulse diagnosis is a key component of acupuncture. When you visit an allopathic doctor's office, the nurse presses lightly on an artery in your wrist and counts the number of times in one minute that the artery "pulses" to determine your heart rate. This seems normal to us because we have grown up with this practice.

Acupuncturists have been using pulse diagnosis for 4,000 years. The practitioner presses on designated locations on your wrists to read distinct pulses on each wrist mirroring the meridians. The acupuncturist is not counting your heart rate. He or she is assessing the quality and quantity of the flow of chi, which provides valuable information. It will indicate where there is blockage in the flow, the extent of the blockage, and if there is imbalance between the left and right sides of your body. In addition to reading your pulse before treatment, the acupuncturist will read it again after the treatment to determine if it was successful in changing the flow of chi.

Based on the pulse diagnosis, the information from the questions, and the acupuncturist's other observations of you, he or she will decide on an appropriate treatment and determine where to place the needles at strategic points along the meridians. You will then lie on the table with the needles for a period of time, allowing them to have an impact.

According to the 2007 National Health Interview Survey, an estimated 3.2 million people in the United States used acupuncture in 2006. Many people seek out acupuncture treatment when Western medical treatments and approaches are not able to help them. Others use it in a complementary or integrative manner in conjunction with Western medical treatment. Acupuncture is popular for addressing chronic conditions, including headaches, allergies, back pain, joint pain, menstrual disorders, anxiety, digestive disorders, sleeping problems, and stress. Acupuncture is also used to address other conditions and as a preventive modality.

Clients of acupuncture have reported having more energy, more vitality, getting sick less often, recovering more quickly when they do get sick, increased mental clarity, and improved emotional well-being. They have also reported the disappearance of ailments or health problems that were not the reason for the initial visit. They claim they are more aware of their body and their symptoms so they can take effective action.

Acupuncture is based on a wellness model that recognizes the natural healing powers of the body, views what is happening within us as a major determinant in disease and illness, and empowers the individual.

HERBS

The use of herbs for their therapeutic or medicinal value is the oldest form of health care. Plants were the first source of medicines. Even animals are observed to use them intuitively for more than simple nourishment. Among plants in any habitat, there are always some with established pharmacological or other medicinal effects. In every rural community since prehistory there were likely to be individuals, most often women, who were regarded as specialists in the art of using plants for healing. They would satisfy the demands of basic health care, including treating injuries and illness. With the move away from the rural community to the city, plants remained the only significant source of medicines and so were transported to the cities.[18]

The ancient Greeks and Romans elaborated herbal concepts that were the basis of Western thought for 1,500 years. The approaches to herbs originating in India and China over 2,000 years ago are still used today.[19]

It has been estimated that up to 75 percent of medicines taken around the world are herbal remedies.[20] The World Health Organization notes that use of herbal medicines is well established and widely acknowledged to be safe and effective.[21]

In most cultures, herbal remedies were traditionally incorporated into a holistic approach to health and wellness. Diseases were viewed as imbalances to be corrected rather than as alien invasions to be attacked. These healing traditions sought to work from within, to find the pattern of disharmony, and to address that disharmony by helping the body heal itself. Herbal remedies were judged by their ability to adjust patterns of disorder, not by any conventional "antidisease" activity.[22]

Herbal medicine is a form of treatment that emphasizes the return to normal balance within the body rather than an attack on symptoms or external agents.[23] Herbal remedies are prescribed specifically with the aim of affecting the behavior of the body and mind, not on attacking a disease.[24] This approach is geared to support the recuperative and defensive self-healing forces of the body.

Some experts in the field believe the success of herbal medicine is based on the total plant rather than on any individual constituent. Plants contain hundreds of constituents. Herbs behave as more than just assemblages of chemicals. When an herbal remedy is examined experimentally, it is typically found to have activity that is apparently more than the sum of its active constituents. Their combination gives it unique properties.[25]

There is a growing interest in herbal medicine and herbal supplements among the general public in Western cultures. In the United States, physicians and health practitioners typically receive little or no training on the topic of herbs. In France and Germany, herbal medicine is taught to doctors as part of their medical training and they prescribe herbs in addition to pharmaceutical drugs.

Consumers are often unclear as to which herbal products will best suit their individual needs and are looking for further guidance. Practitioners who are educated in the properties of herbs and have received training in their uses can be a valuable resource in the health care field.

There is not one right way to address health and wellness concerns, as evidenced by the practices of different cultures across the planet and across time. Shifting your perspective to include an awareness of various wellness modalities gives you the opportunity to do further research and to consider new possibilities in addressing your unique health care situation and needs.

REFLECTIONS

⌒⊗⌒

THE SAMURAI

Once upon a time, a towering samurai warrior approached a small Zen monk. "Teach me about heaven and hell!" the samurai growled.

"Teach you?" the monk responded. "You are a dirty, smelly, unkempt poor excuse for a samurai. Even your sword is rusty!"

The samurai, stung to the quick, flushed with anger and, in an instant, drew his sword, raising it high so as to cleave the insolent monk in two. A split second before the sword began its downward arc, the monk pointed and said, "That's Hell!"

A flash of insight washed over the samurai. This little monk, he thought, had gone to the brink of death to teach him. The samurai's body relaxed and a sense of gratitude welled up in him as he sheathed his sword. At that very moment, the monk said, "That's Heaven!"[26]

A CUP OF TEA

A wise Zen master was well respected and people came from all over to learn from him and seek his wisdom. One day he was visited by an educated man who considered himself an expert in Zen. The visitor indicated he was quite knowledgeable already and wanted to speak with the master just in case there was anything he had missed.

The Zen master said they should discuss it over a cup of tea. The master poured the visitor a cup. He kept pouring until the tea spilled over the cup and onto the visitor's lap. The visitor shouted at the master, "What are you doing? Can't you see the cup is full?"

The master stopped pouring and smiled at his guest. "You are like this tea cup, so full of ideas and opinions that nothing more can be added. Come back to me when the cup is empty, with an empty mind. Then you will learn."

❦

In order to change we must be sick and tired of being sick and tired.

~UNKNOWN

Not everything that can be counted counts and not everything that counts can be counted.

~ALBERT EINSTEIN

People have a hard time letting go of their suffering. Out of a fear of the unknown, they prefer suffering that is familiar.

~THICH NHAT HANH

Our finest moments are more likely to occur when we are feeling deeply uncomfortable, unhappy or unfulfilled. For it is only in such moments, propelled by discomfort, that we are likely to step out of our ruts and start searching for different ways or truer answers.

~M. SCOTT PECK

Doctors and scientists said that breaking the four minute mile was impossible, that one would die in the attempt. Thus when I got up from the track after collapsing at the finish line, I figured I was dead.

~ROGER BANISTER

*The marvelous pharmacy that was designed by nature
and placed into our being by the universal architect
produces most of the medicines that we need.*

~NORMAN COUSINS

*Stop the mindless wishing that things would be different. Rather than
wasting time and emotional and spiritual energy in explaining why we
don't have what we want, we can start to pursue other ways to get it.*

~GREG ANDERSON

*It is a common theme in the folklore of the Arabian Nights
that when you stumble and fall there you find the gold.*

~JOSEPH CAMPBELL

*If you look deeply into the palm of your hand, you will see
your parents and all generations of your ancestors. All of
them are alive in this moment. Each is present in your body.
You are the continuation of each of these people.*

~THICH NHAT HANH

*Always listen to experts. They'll tell you what
can't be done and why. Then do it.*

~ROBERT HEINLEIN

*The real voyage of discovery rests not in seeking
new landscapes, but in having new eyes.*

~MARCEL PROUST

You miss 100% of the shots you don't take.

~WAYNE GRETZKY

SHIFT 7

Partnership

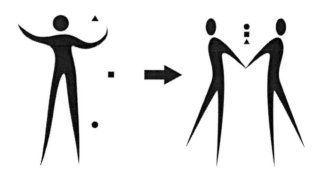

CHAPTER 7

Shift 7: PARTNERSHIP

Shift: You are impacting the health and wellness of others.

We not only impact our own health and wellness, each of us is impacting the health and wellness of others. It doesn't matter that we may not be intending to have an impact. What we say and do most definitely makes a difference and has health and wellness implications. How would we speak and act differently if we could see the health impact our words and actions were having on others? Shifting your perspective to recognize that you are in fact "a wellness practitioner" directly influencing the health and wellness of others each day may result in a shift in your actions.

HEALING PRESENCE

Here is a powerful phrase you likely have never heard: "Be a healing presence."[1] What does it mean to be a healing presence or to be a practitioner of wellness? The terms "practitioner" and "healing" apply in a broader context than just that of the traditional medical framework.

A practitioner is typically defined as one who engages in or practices a trained occupation or profession. Within a medical context a practitioner is someone you go to for a treatment of some kind to improve your health or wellness. This could be a physician, an acupuncturist, an herbalist, a chiropractor, an optometrist, or a massage therapist. To be a practitioner implies consciously taking action with the intent of helping others. Yet, each of us impacts the health, wellness and well-being of others by our words and actions even if we are not intending to have that impact.

"Healing" is also a broader concept than that assumed in the traditional medical context. Healing is typically defined as the process of restoring to health. Taking a wider view supports the concept of being a healing presence. Being a healing presence is to have your presence, through your actions and speech, have a positive impact on others. Being a healing presence is to act or speak in a manner that brings more possibility into someone's life. Being a healing presence is to create conditions in which there is less unnecessary suffering.

Being a healing presence can also be looked at in a more literal sense. We know that some diseases or illnesses are contagious. Being contagious means that you transmit the disease germs that have invaded your body to someone else's body, who then gets sick.

Consider that wellness and well-being are also contagious—that our presence can "infect" others and affect their mood and their health and well-being. What happens when you're having a great day and you walk around in an upbeat mood? Do other people tend to become positive and upbeat when they are around you? What happens when you're in a grumpy, complaining, pessimistic mood? Do the people around you reflect your mood and behavior? What happens to your own mood when you encounter someone who is upbeat and positive, or grumpy and complaining? You know from personal experience that moods are contagious.

Remember the saying, "One rotten apple spoils the whole barrel"? The rotten part of one apple spreads throughout the barrel because it infects not only the apples it touches but gets passed on from apple to apple until all the apples are infected. The same process applies to people. We can not only spread germs and illnesses but also our moods and way of being.

Life around us shows up differently because of our presence. What we say and do and how we are affects others and has a direct impact on their health, wellness and well-being.

The concept of being a healing presence serves as a powerful reminder of both the opportunity and responsibility we all have. You may not have thought of it in these terms, but you have been, currently are, and will continue to be a magnificent healing presence.

LANGUAGE AS "TREATMENT"

We each have the power to impact someone else's health, wellness and well-being through the words we say. We may not think about it and may take it for granted but it is an absolute fact. Each of us has the opportunity to administer a "wellness treatment" to many people every day if we choose.

As kids, we learned the saying, "Sticks and stones may break my bones but words will never hurt me." It's not true. Words can have a more profound and longer lasting impact then getting hit with sticks and stones. The upside of words over sticks and stones is that words can have a positive as well as a negative impact.

Mind and body are connected. If you have a negative impact on the mind, it will show up as a negative impact in your body. Words can not only cause psychological and emotional damage, they can also cause physical damage. The reverse is also true. If you have a positive impact on the mind, it will show up as a positive impact in your body.

If you tell a child he is stupid, your words will impact his wellness and well-being. Your language will influence how he feels about himself and what he expects from himself. It will impact how he feels about you. It will impact his happiness. These effects will show up in his body in some way. Calling a child stupid will have a profound and long-lasting impact on his wellness and well-being.

If you tell a child he is smart, that too will impact his wellness and well-being. It will influence how he feels about himself, what he expects from himself, and how he feels about you. It will impact his happiness. It will show up in his body in some way. Calling a child smart will have a profound and long-lasting effect on his wellness and well-being.

If you say thank you to a relative, coworker, friend or stranger for something they gave you or some service they provided, you will have a positive impact on their wellness and well-being. There will be a physical change in the person's body as a result of your acknowledgment of them. It may have a prolonged or only a momentary effect, but it will definitely have an impact. You will have made a difference in that person's life, even if only for a moment or a day.

Think of how you respond to words that are spoken to you and how they affect your response to a situation. Think of situations in the last week where you would have chosen different words if you had considered their impact on the health and wellness of the other person.

All day long we interact and have conversations with other people: family members, friends, colleagues and strangers. What we say and how we say it will have an impact on the health and wellness of those people because their body will react in some way. Consider what you would say differently if you consciously thought, "What I am about to say will impact this person's health either positively or negatively."

The flip side is that other people are hurling words at you all day as well. Some of them will be coming at you like sticks and stones. The good news is you have a choice about whether or not they hurt you. If you choose to let them hurt you, you also have a choice as to how deeply and for how long they hurt you and how you will relate to them.

Here is a practice you can do to see for yourself the power you have. Every day for the next week give at least one person an acknowledgment. It can be a thank you, it can be noticing something they did, it can be recognizing something they achieved, or it can be complimenting them on their clothes. An acknowledgment is essentially telling the person, "I know you are here and there is something positive about you."

We all long for acknowledgment. As you're acknowledging someone, observe the reaction you get. Observe their body. Observe how it appears to make them feel. Observe how it makes you feel. Observe what shows up in your body. Observe what shows up in your thoughts and emotions. Observe how this person interacts with you the next time you see them. Observe how it affects your relationship with them.

The concept that words matter may seem obvious. You may be thinking, "It's no big deal. Of course what I say has an impact," or "It's obvious that I'll get a different reaction from someone if I'm nasty rather than nice." My intention in highlighting this concept is to point to the fact that we can make a conscious choice about what impact we're going to have on another person's health and wellness through our language and actions. We live in a sea of words. They pour down on us like rain all day long and have much more of an impact than most of us ever consider.

The world changes as a result of our speaking. Life shows up differently based on what we say and how we say it. Each of us is a wellness practitioner who is impacting the health of those we interact with.

What a wonderful opportunity to make a positive difference in the lives of others by being conscious of the words we speak.

THE YIN YANG OF RELATIONSHIPS

Yin yang is a key concept in Chinese philosophy, culture, and medicine. It illustrates a major distinction between a Western view of life and an Eastern view.

In Western philosophy and culture we think of things that are opposite as being separate and distinct from one another. Examples are good/evil, day/night, active/passive, north/south, positive/negative, winter/summer, male/female, light/dark, hot/cold, white/black. This is a dualistic view in which opposites are mutually exclusive and either one or the other exists.

The Chinese view is based on the principle of polarity, where opposites are complementary and coexist within a cycle of movement from one to the other.[2] Both exist at the same time, with one aspect manifesting more than the other at any given moment. The opposites are united as a whole and depend upon each other. There cannot be north without south, inside without outside, positive without negative.

Yin and yang represent the fundamental opposites and polarities of the universe, where there is a continuous balancing act and movement between the two aspects. Any pair of opposites is believed to have a polar relationship where each of the two poles is linked to and dependent on the other. The opposites are in tension but they complement and balance one another, with neither aspect of more importance than the other. The yin and yang model is used to describe how opposing forces are interdependent and interconnected in the natural world. Life is the blended harmony of the two polarities.

The conception of yin and yang grew from the observation of nature.

Yin originally referred to the shady side of the mountain and was associated with cold. Yang referred to the sunny side and was associated with warmth and light. As the sun moves across the sky, yin and yang gradually trade places with each other and the process repeats itself. The concept of yin and yang is extended to apply to everything in the universe, whereby everything has both yin and yang aspects which are constantly interacting.

The yin yang symbol below illustrates this concept. The black and white shapes represent the interaction of two energies or forces, the yin and yang. The circle represents the universe. The shapes are complementary and balance one another within the circle. The shape of the yin and yang sections gives a sense of movement of these two energies. There is not a beginning or an end. Day does not suddenly become night; there is a gradual movement from one to the other, and then the cycle repeats itself.

The two dots in the black and white shapes symbolize that each of the two energies or forces contains the seed of its polar opposite. Even when one of the forces reaches its extreme it still contains within itself the seed of its opposite.

In the yin yang symbol, the black section represents yin, which is associated with the qualities of darkness, cold, inward and downward direction, rest, inhibition, femaleness, slowness, softness, wetness, night, and tranquility. Yang is represented by the white section and is associated with brightness, heat, outward and upward direction, movement, activity and excitement, maleness, speed, hardness, dryness, daytime, and aggressiveness.

Yin and yang represent all the opposite principles that exist in the universe, and no one principle continually dominates the other. There is a cycle, with constant movement and balancing between the opposing principles. Opposites that we experience—health and sickness, wealth and poverty, strength and softness—can be explained by the temporary dominance of one principle over the other. Since no one principle dominates eternally, all conditions are subject to change into their opposites and have the seeds of their opposites within them. For example, sickness has the seeds of health and health contains the seeds of sickness. Even though an opposite may not be seen or appear to be present, it is in fact there. We are not totally healthy or totally sick but embody both qualities at the same time.

Chinese medicine is based on the principle of achieving a proper balance between yin and yang. When you are sick or ill, you are out of balance. Actions that you and a practitioner take are aimed at helping your body return to a state of proper balance.

The yin yang principle can also be applied to relationships. We all have many relationships. In our families we have relationships such as mother/daughter, mother/son, husband/wife, father/son, father/daughter, sister/brother, and so forth. Work-setting relationships include employee/manager, salesperson/customer, colleague/colleague, manager/staff. We have relationships with people we are dating and with friends, neighbors, acquaintances, and strangers.

Relationships flourish when there is collaboration and partnership between the people involved. When the yin and yang factors are out of balance, there is disharmony.

There are a number of models that characterize relationships. In one, the individuals focus on their separateness, whereby one person is more important than the other or the relationship.[3] In this approach my wants and needs are what count. As long as I get what I want, the relationship doesn't matter. It's about me winning. If I win, then you must lose. This attitude upsets the balance of yin and yang and may cause disharmony in a relationship.

Another relationship style is for one person to focus on the wants and needs of the other. In this approach, my attention is on making you happy, regardless of its impact on me or on the relationship. The focus is on you winning and me losing and about catering to your needs at the expense of my own. This approach also upsets the balance of yin and yang and may cause disharmony.

A third option is to create a partnership in which each person chooses to act in ways that are best for the relationship rather than to benefit one party at the expense of the other. Decisions are made for the sake of the relationship/partnership, which flourishes along with the people involved. The yin and yang are in balance, and harmony in the relationship is achieved.

As in nature and in the yin and yang model, there is movement in relationships. There is an ongoing balancing that is taking place. Just as the yin and yang make up the whole, there are two sides to all issues and situations in relationships. When there is imbalance between the two people involved, disharmony occurs. Finding the proper balance between the two sides and resolving issues brings the relationship back into harmony.

Think of relationships you have and the ups and downs you experience within them. What is out of balance during the down times? What is the dominating principle or characteristic? What is in balance during the up times? What is the nature of the relationship when there is a commitment to partnership rather than to individual gain?

You can call upon your observer to reflect upon your relationships and then create movement or a shift toward greater balance within them. However, the yin yang concept reminds us that relationships are not static but are fluid and moving. They will not remain permanently in balance and harmony, but will go through natural cycles. The good news is that balance and harmony can reoccur if action is taken to move in that direction.

Each of us is in a health and wellness partnership with others. Shifting your viewpoint to focus on the impact you are having on someone else's health and wellness will likely result in a shift in your words and actions.

REFLECTIONS

⤸

THE ONE-EYED MONK

In ancient times traveling monks when arriving at a monastery could challenge the monks to a theological contest and would be given food and shelter if they won but would have to go to the next monastery if they lost. There was a monastery occupied by two brothers, a wise monk with two eyes and a not-so-smart monk with one eye. One night it was raining very hard and a traveling monk knocked on the door. The wise brother, wishing to be kind to the wet monk, suggested he have a contest with his less skilled brother. The traveling monk proceeded to the other room to challenge the brother.

Five minutes later the contest was over. The traveling monk entered the room, bowed and admitted defeat. The wise brother said, "Tell me what happened." The traveling monk replied, "Your brother is a genius." He continued, "We decided to debate in silence. I went first and held up one finger, signifying the Buddha. Your brother held up two fingers, meaning the Buddha and his teachings. I replied with three fingers, indicating the Buddha, his teachings and his followers. Your brother replied in brilliance when he showed me his fist proving that in reality the Buddha, his teachings, and his followers are all one."

The monk bowed once more and went on his way on the stormy

night. Just then the brother entered and was very irate. "That man was so rude. If he was not our guest I would have thrown him out of our monastery." "What happened?" the wise brother asked. The one-eyed brother replied, "We decided to have a silent debate and the first thing he did was hold up one finger, meaning, 'I see you have only one eye.' So I held up two fingers out of courtesy to him, meaning 'I see you have two eyes.' But the traveler was so rude, he held up three fingers, telling me that together the two of us have only three eyes. I lost my temper and I shook my fist at him and he left the room."

A PRICELESS SACK

Mulla came upon a frowning man walking along the road to town. "What's wrong?" he asked. The man held up a tattered bag and moaned, "All that I own in this wide world barely fills this miserable, wretched sack."

"Too bad," said Mulla, and with that he snatched the bag from the man's hand and ran down the road with it.

Having lost everything, the man burst into tears and more miserable than before continued walking. Meanwhile, Mulla quickly ran around the bend and placed the man's sack in the middle of the road, where he would have to come upon it. When the man saw his bag sitting in the road before him he laughed with joy and shouted, "My sack! I thought I had lost you!"

Watching through the bushes, Mulla chuckled, "Well, that's one way to make someone happy!"[4]

Words are, of course, the most powerful drugs used by mankind.
~RUDYARD KIPLING

Watch your thoughts because they become your words; Watch your words because they become your habits; Watch your habits because they become your character; Watch your character because it becomes your destiny.
~PLATO

One word determines the whole world.
~ZEN SAYING

It is the enemy who can truly teach us to practice the virtues of compassion and tolerance.
~THE DALAI LAMA

If you treat an individual as he is, he will stay as he is. But if you treat him as if he were what he ought to be and could be, he will become what he ought to be and what he could be.
~JOHANN WOLFGANG VON GOETHE

We can't do great things; we can only do small things with great love.
~MOTHER TERESA

Act as if what you do makes a difference. It does.
~WILLIAM JAMES

Words have the power to both destroy and heal. When words are both true and kind they can change our world.
~BUDDHA

One of the noblest words in our language is grace, defined as "unearned blessing." We live by grace far more than by anything else. Accordingly . . . one thing I want to put into practice in my own life is the conscious and deliberate habit of finding somebody to thank.
~ELTON TRUEBLOOD

Be kind; everyone you meet is fighting a hard battle.

~JOHN WATSON

Feeling gratitude and not expressing it is like wrapping a present and not giving it.

~WILLIAM ARTHUR WARD

Out beyond ideas of wrongdoing and rightdoing, there is a field. I'll meet you there.

~RUMI

Words lead to deeds . . . They prepare the soul, make it ready, and move it to tenderness.

~MOTHER TERESA

Service

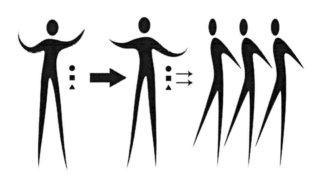

CHAPTER 8

Shift 8: SERVICE

Shift: You possess enormous ability and have the opportunity
to impact the wellness and well-being of the world.

Not only can you impact your own health and wellness, you
have the talent, skills, qualities and experience to impact the
wellness and well-being of the world. We are all making a difference
in the health and wellness of our family, our loved ones, and people
with whom we come in direct contact. Those people touch other people,
who touch other people, who touch other people. The impact we have
on one person spreads and impacts others, and we do not know the
rippled ramifications of our actions. Impacting the world is not limited
to taking some action on a global issue such as the elimination of world
hunger. Impacting the wellness of the world can start with being a positive influence on how life shows up around you. Impacting the wellness
of the world includes being a healing presence that reduces unnecessary
suffering. Shifting to a recognition that every day you have an opportunity to impact the wellness of the world will make a difference in many
lives.

YOU ARE A LEADER

You are a leader. Even if you don't think of yourself as a leader, you have leadership skills and talents that you use every day. You are so good at being a leader, you do it instinctively.

Every day you have the opportunity to use your leadership skills to improve the wellness and well-being of others. You have the potential to learn more skills and tools to increase your effectiveness and impact as a leader.

Many people have a very narrow view or definition of a leader. Some think of a leader as a person who is designated as being in charge of a group of people. A leader is frequently thought to be someone who has superiority or control over others. Leaders might include a general in the military, a governor, a department head in a company, the head of the PTA, the owner of a company, the den mother of a Girl Scout troop, a manager of a baseball team, a conductor of an orchestra, a manager of a store, a school principal, a head of an organization, a foreman, a manager of a department.

Think of the people who are traditionally considered leaders. What is it they do as leaders? They may be in charge of people or projects. They may make decisions that impact others in their area of control. They may plan. They may respond to situations. They may be responsible for seeing that action is taken. They may consider the impact of their action on others. They may have others looking to them for guidance or support. They may have a desire or passion to bring about change or make something happen.

You do not have to be designated and identified as the leader to have an impact and exhibit leadership qualities. Think about your life and how many times the above actions apply to what you do during a week.

Being a parent involves leadership. There are family situations that occur when you are a leader and employ leadership skills. Organizing the breakfast menu for your family is demonstrating leadership. Leading a discussion and planning on where to go for a vacation is leadership. Coordinating your children's activities is leadership. Resolving disputes between your kids is leadership. Taking care of your parents is a sign of leadership. Finding and buying a house for your family is leadership. Taking action to resolve a disagreement with your spouse is leadership. Counseling and advising a family member is leadership.

There are work situations in which you employ leadership skills. Resolving disputes among coworkers is leadership. Taking an action to improve morale is leadership. Volunteering to perform a task is leadership. Not participating in office gossip is leadership. Training or helping coworkers is leadership. Listening and providing support to a coworker who is experiencing suffering in his or her life is leadership.

There are situations with strangers when you exhibit leadership. Helping someone by holding a door open is leadership. Offering a compliment to someone working in a store is leadership. Performing volunteer work is leadership.

Here are some competencies and capabilities of leaders as they traditionally relate to business situations: organizing, motivating, taking charge, inspiring others, managing change, problem solving, making decisions, planning, teaching and coaching others, communicating clearly, allocating tasks, listening and providing feedback, caring for others, delegating, achieving results, building trust and cooperation, doing the right thing, setting goals. Here are some characteristics frequently ascribed to leaders: honesty, resilience, resourcefulness, flexibility, fair-mindedness, humor.

Think about these characteristics and competencies and about how often you exhibit these same qualities on a daily basis by merely living your life. You are performing leadership actions every day even if you don't think of yourself as being a leader.

Leadership can be based on interrelationship and collaboration rather than on having superiority over others. "You can lead from any seat"[1] without being the designated leader or person in charge.

You can use the skills and techniques outlined in this book to be a more effective leader in any relationship and in all aspects of your life. You can use your leadership talents and qualities to have a positive impact on the wellness and well-being of the world.

SEVEN GENERATIONS

The Navajo have a saying that suggests an individual has a responsibility to seven generations. According to this teaching, each of us stands in the midst of seven generations: the three generations that preceded you—your parents, grandparents, and great-grandparents—and the three generations that will follow you: your children, grandchildren, and great-grandchildren. The seventh generation is your current generation.[2]

Applying this principle means we have a responsibility to honor our ancestors and serve our children. We as individuals have a responsibility beyond our individual selves. In decisions we make and actions we take we should ask ourselves two fundamental questions: Will this honor my parents and their parents and their parents? Will this serve my children, their children, and their children?

Another way of looking at it is: Would my ancestors be proud of the action I am taking? What impact does my action have on the life my children, grandchildren, and great-grandchildren will lead?

This concept of honoring the ancestors and serving the children is not unique to the Navajo. Wisdom traditions from around the world have similar philosophies about honoring, respecting, and learning from elders and about having a responsibility to act for the benefit of future generations rather than only for oneself.

This may sound like a rather obvious principle, but it is extremely powerful. How many of us would act differently on a daily basis if we evaluated our actions against the criterion, does it honor the ancestors and serve the children?

Imagine the impact if, when considering our personal well-being, our relationships with friends and relatives, or our actions at work, we asked not "What do I feel like doing?" or "What would make me happy?" but "What action at this moment will honor my parents, grandparents, and great-grandparents and will serve not only my children but my grandchildren and great-grandchildren?"[3]

Think of how you can apply this principle to your own life. Think of situations that occurred in the past week and how you may have acted differently if you had applied this principle. Think of relationships you have and how you would like to alter them based on applying this principle.

POWER TO MAKE AN IMPACT

One of the major themes of this book is that you have the power to control your own health, wellness and well-being. You can choose to take action if you decide it will serve you. This may require making changes from your normal way of behaving, and it will require practice. The changes you make may feel uncomfortable or strange or out of your comfort zone or totally opposite from how you see yourself.

Remember that you are very practiced at thinking, acting, behaving, and feeling a certain way and that you are a beginner at the new approach you have chosen. You are fully capable of applying anything covered in this book if you choose to do it. It may require practice, but you can do it.

Another theme of this book is that you have the power to make an impact on the health, wellness and well-being of others. Every day you have the power to impact your family, friends, coworkers, strangers, community, and your world. There are things you can do and actions you can take to make a positive impact on others. You can use the information and materials in this book to serve others if you so choose.

Shifting to a recognition that you possess enormous leadership ability and have an opportunity to impact the wellness and well-being of the world will make a difference in your actions. You are encouraged to use the concepts, ideas, and distinctions in this book to make a difference and to share the knowledge, insights, and wisdom you have gained with others.

REFLECTIONS

⚍

STARFISH

Strolling along the edge of the sea, a man catches sight of a young woman who appears to be engaged in a ritual dance. She stoops down, then straightens to her full height, casting her arm out in an arc. Drawing closer he sees that the beach around her is littered with starfish, and she is throwing them one by one into the sea. He lightly mocks her: "There are stranded starfish as far as the eye can see, for miles up the beach. What difference can saving a few of them possibly make?" Smiling, she bends down and once more tosses a starfish out over the water, saying serenely, "It certainly makes a difference to this one."[4]

HEAVEN AND HELL

A woman who had worked all her life to bring about good was granted one wish: "Before I die let me visit both hell and heaven." Her wish was granted.

She was whisked off to a great banqueting hall. The tables were piled high with delicious food and drink. Around the table sat miserable starving people. "Why are they like this?" she asked the angel who accompanied her. "Look at their arms," the angel replied. She looked and saw that attached to each person's arms were five-feet-long chopsticks secured above the elbow. Unable to bend their elbows, the people were repeatedly unable to pick up the food and put it in their mouths. They sat hungry, frustrated and miserable. "This is clearly hell," said the woman.

She was then whisked off to heaven. She found herself in an identical banquet hall with tables piled high with delicious food and drink. Around the tables sat people laughing, contented and joyful. She noticed that the people had five-feet-long chopsticks secured above the elbow just as in hell. The difference was here everyone was serving the person across the table and they all became abundantly full.[5]

≈

To find our calling is to find the intersection between our
own deep gladness and the world's deep hunger.
~Frederick Buechner

How far you go in life depends on your being tender with the young,
compassionate with the aged, sympathetic with the striving, and tolerant
of the weak and strong. Because someday you will have been all of these.
~George Washington Carver

We are unified with all life that is nature. Man can
no longer live his life for himself alone.
~Albert Schweitzer

Knowing is not enough; we must apply. Willing is not enough; we must do.
~Johann Wolfgang von Goethe

It is one of the most beautiful compensations of this life that you
cannot sincerely try to help another without helping yourself.
~Ralph Waldo Emerson

We do not inherit the earth from our ancestors,
we borrow it from our children.
~NATIVE AMERICAN PROVERB

The more you lose yourself in something bigger than
yourself, the more energy you will have.
~NORMAN VINCENT PEALE

Never doubt that a small group of thoughtful, committed citizens
can change the world. Indeed, it is the only thing that ever has.
~MARGARET MEAD

Remember, if you need a helping hand, you'll find one at the end
of your arm . . . As you grow older you will discover that you have
two hands. One for helping yourself, the other for helping others.
~AUDREY HEPBURN

I don't know what your destiny will be, but one thing I
know: The only ones among you who will be truly happy are
those who will have sought and found how to serve.
~ALBERT SCHWEITZER

From what we get, we can make a living; what
we give, however, makes a life.
~ARTHUR ASHE

To laugh often and much, to win the respect of intelligent people and the
affection of children . . . to leave the world a bit better . . . to know even one
life has breathed easier because you have lived, this is to have succeeded.
~RALPH WALDO EMERSON

Service is the rent that you pay for room on this earth.
~SHIRLEY CHISHOLM

We must be the change we wish to see in the world.
~MAHATMA GANDHI

Practices

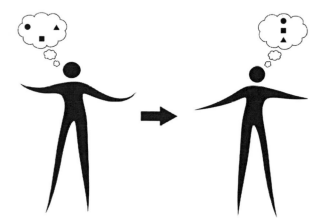

CHAPTER 9

PRACTICES

I f you want to learn to play the piano, you can begin by reading books about theory and about how to play and where to place your fingers. However, to learn to actually play the piano you must apply that information by sitting at the piano, placing your fingers on the keys, and pressing them. Being a beginner, at first you may think it is difficult, but if you wish to improve, you will need to sit at the piano and repeatedly practice. No matter how much theoretical knowledge you have, without practice you will never learn to play the piano.

At first you will need to think about where to place your fingers and what key to hit and how long to hold the note and which key is next. After you practice for a period of time your fingers may automatically move to the correct key without your thinking so much. It becomes more instinctive. This is an example of embodied learning. The learning is becoming part of you in such a way that you act instinctively.

The more you practice, the better you get at playing. As you become better at hitting the keys, you may start to work with the foot pedals. You practice and practice, and after a while you are playing the keys you want and using the pedals to create the beautiful music you desire. It just flows from you. You can almost feel the music in your body. Your learning has become part of you. Mozart, Beethoven and all the great pianists of the world started out just like you: by being a beginner and sitting down at the piano for the first time having never played before.

You can speak about "being a beginner" as opposed to something being hard or difficult.[1] We have learned to act or be a certain way throughout our life and we are comfortable with it because we are practiced at acting or thinking that way. Making a change may appear to be hard or uncomfortable only because we are not as practiced at acting or thinking the new way. We are beginners. We have learned to act or think a certain way over many years, and we can learn to act or think a different way by practicing doing it differently.

Learning to drive a car is another example of something that appeared to be hard at first because you were just a beginner. You had to learn the mechanics of driving and think about your actions. After repeated practice it became embodied learning, and now you drive instinctively without consciously thinking about each aspect of the process.

The information this book contains provides you with an opportunity to impact your health and wellness and that of others in positive ways. But similar to reading about how to play the piano or how to drive a car, reading the information is only valuable if that information is applied and practiced. You may be very practiced at some of the concepts covered in this book, while in other areas you may be a beginner.

The more any of the concepts and teachings are put to use, the more they will become embodied in you. Specific practices are provided at the end of the chapter to assist you in applying some of these concepts and ideas. The idea behind a practice is that you wake up in the morning with the intention to consciously apply it. You look for situations during the day—at home and work; with family, friends or strangers—in which you can apply the practice. Just as in practicing the piano, the more you practice the recommended thinking and behaviors, the more comfortable you will become with acting and thinking in a new way.

You can pick a particular practice and apply it every day for four or five days. As you apply the practice, observe how it makes your body feel, how it makes you feel emotionally, how it impacts your sense of wellness and well-being, how other people react to you, how the practice impacts someone else's wellness and well-being, how it impacts a relationship. Note any shifts that occur as you apply the practice. Observe how life shows up differently based on your actions or words. Compare this to how you would typically have acted in this situation and the impact it would have had on you and others.

In addition to the practices listed, you may want to come up with some of your own. You may want to repeat a practice. You will find that you will have opportunities throughout each day to use more than one of the practices, and that is fantastic. Apply the information you have learned whenever it serves you or others to do so.

- Have your observer present in a situation in which you would normally just react unconsciously.
- Choose "Upset is optional" in a situation.
- Add five minutes of additional exercise or movement in the middle of the day.
- Choose large mind.
- Do something unexpected for someone.
- Let go of a squawk for one day for the sake of someone.
- Acknowledge someone. Fill the day with acknowledgment.

- Discontinue for one week eating something you know is un-healthy for you.
- Look for an opening to improve a relationship and take some appropriate action.
- Choose your mood first thing in the morning and see how it affects others.
- Take an additional five-minute break during the day.
- Be a leader in a situation in which you would not normally lead.
- Act rather than react in a situation.
- Recognize when you are creating a story rather than observing the phenomena and create a larger, more useful story.
- Notice a symptom and determine what you can learn from it.
- Find an opportunity to be a healing presence.
- Use your breathing to assist you in relating to a situation.
- Accept a situation for what it is rather than trying to change it.
- Share something you learned with someone.
- Spend five minutes in peaceful stillness or meditation.
- Allow yourself to be a beginner in a situation that you think is difficult.
- Take some effective action to address any stress you are experiencing.
- Give a verbal gift to someone.
- When experiencing a problem or crisis, ask yourself, "What is the opportunity here?"
- Do something new to honor the ancestors.
- Observe your body to notice or learn something new.
- Communicate gratitude. Fill the day with gratitude.
- Take three deep breaths throughout the day.
- Offer assistance to someone.

- Perform an act that you would not usually do and that you can declare is a contribution.
- Call or talk to someone you have not spoken to for a while.
- Do something new for the sake of the next generations.
- Practice genuinely listening to others and speaking less.
- Do something nice for a total stranger.
- Give a gift (not necessarily something that costs money) to someone based on what you think that person would love to receive.

Conclusion

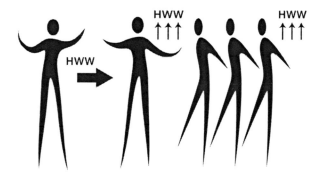

CHAPTER 10

CONCLUSION

W ow! That was a lot to take in. New information, new ways of looking at old information, new shifts, new ways of thinking and acting, stories and quotes, concepts and distinctions, comparing and contrasting different approaches to wellness, awakening to new powers, unusual analogies, new choices and possibilities, acknowledging that you have the ability to directly impact others' wellness and well-being, stick figure drawings, and practices. It could easily make your head spin and have you become overwhelmed.

Let me help. The information and material in this book is not a linear and rigid program whereby you need to implement each of the shifts, concepts or practices and apply them in a specified sequence to enhance your health, wellness, and well-being. You can implement or embrace just one idea in this book and create a better world for you, your loved ones, and others.

The book started with the analogy of having a meal with friends at a popular restaurant called Fusion. It specialized in fusion cuisine which combines elements of various traditions from different countries and cultures from around the world. The four-course meal was designed to introduce you to new possibilities in cooking, just as the book is intended to introduce you to new options in approaching health and wellness.

Now that you have been introduced to these new possibilities and had a taste of their potential to enhance your life, let me give you a new analogy that may be helpful in moving forward. Think of the book as providing you with powerful tools and an instruction manual for using those tools to make a positive change in your life. You may choose to reacquaint yourself with all the tools and then decide which ones to use and at what speed and intensity to use them. Keep in mind that it can be quite invigorating and rewarding to use tools that you are not accustomed to handling.

I encourage you to start with shift 1, Reframing, and shift 2, Empowerment, because they establish an important framework for viewing health and wellness. From that knowledge base, pick another shift or practice that resonates with you. Reread the appropriate section and choose a practice to implement for four days and see what shows up. Then choose another concept and practice for the next four days, while also being aware of the first practice, to see if there are situations in which you can use it. Then choose other concepts to embrace and practice. Embodied learning will occur best when you consciously take action to implement a change from your default settings.

As you live each day, look for opportunities to use the material from the book. At the end of the day, think about situations you encountered in which concepts, distinctions, or practices from the book may have been useful. What you discover may be a good starting point for selecting which tools you want to pick up first.

The book was designed to be a valuable resource that you may want to reread and refer to as you make shifts. There is nothing in it that is overly complex and complicated or outside of your abilities to use if you so choose. In fact, that's one of the beauties of these eight shifts and the material presented. The drawings used to illustrate the shifts were intentionally done with stick figures because they reflect the fact that the shifts, concepts, distinctions and practices are easily understood, can be universally applied, and can be powerful without being complicated or complex. You can also use the stick figure drawings to explain the shifts to others.

One of the goals of the book is to encourage you to rethink your own role in affecting your health, wellness, and well-being. Another is to inspire you to take action. To that end I offer one more tool: a reminding fable.

Imagine a magical village where the people and animals live in harmony. In this land there are many different kinds of animals that are much different than the animals you and I are accustomed to seeing. Some have wings or six legs or unusual features or unusual talents. The animals wander around interacting with the villagers in a peaceful coexistence.

The people of this village live a good life. They work and play and have relationships and families. They experience sorrow and misfortune and complications in their lives but are able to deal with them and for the most part are happy. For most of them, their health, wellness, and well-being (HWW) is at an acceptable level, although some have a level that is higher than average and others want to increase their level.

In this village there is a very special animal called a *reac* (pronounced ree-ack) that has four legs, a tail, wings, and big floppy ears which it uses to frequently cover its mouth. Reacs freely walk around the village and come in contact with the villagers. Some villagers just ignore them, while others pay attention to their every move.

You see, the reac has unique powers. A reac has the ability to increase the HWW level of any villager. More specifically, the lips of the reac have this ability. In this magical land the villagers spell differently than we do, and lips is spelled *lpps*. The lips of the reac look basic and simple and unspectacular. However, their powers cannot be denied. If a villager is exposed to the lips of a reac, his or her HWW level will increase. The longer and more frequent the exposure, the greater the impact.

Some villagers are very aware of the powerful nature of the reac lips and they study and track the animal to find a time when it uncovers its mouth. These villagers are very focused on increasing their HWW level and look for every opportunity to get exposure to the reac lips and try to actually embrace them. Other villagers are not aware of the power of the reac lips and therefore take no action. The villagers are all happy and doing the best they can, and at the same time they each have an opportunity to increase their HWW level.

In order to remember the eight shifts, think of the magical powers of the ree-ack lips – *REAC LPPS.*

Reframing
Empowerment
Awakening
Choices

Living
Possibilities
Partnership
Service

While it may never become a classic teaching story, this fable is quirky enough to stick with you, and I can tell you from personal experience that REAC LPPS is a great way to remember the eight shifts.

At the end of this chapter is a recap of the eight shifts and the drawings. These can also serve to help you remember and embrace the shifts.

I honestly believe the eight shifts and "reac lips" are game changers which will enhance both your life and the world in a substantial way. You don't need to implement all of the shifts to have a noticeable impact on your life. Implement any one of the shifts and it will rock your wellness world. Here is a little experiment. Every day for the next two weeks say "eight shifts reac lips" as a reminder to yourself. See how life shows up differently for you and around you. I think you will be amazed.

I hope that you are inspired to not only make shifts in your own life, but also share the information with others so they can make shifts in their lives. Similar to the experience of a group of friends or family eating at the Fusion restaurant, the concepts, principles, and shifts that resonated with you may not be the same ones that resonate with your friends and family. Therefore, I encourage you to not only share the information with others but share the book as well so they can discover for themselves the potential for new possibilities in their lives.

There is old saying that if you give a person a fish you feed him or her for a day and if you teach a person to fish you feed him or her for a lifetime. I have an expansion on this saying. "Teach a person to fish and inspire him or her to teach others to fish and you will feed a village for a lifetime." The material in the book will hopefully enhance your fishing for a lifetime and inspire you to share the information with others.

There are many ways the material in this book can be used to enhance your life and the lives of others. I am interested in hearing how you have used the material and in sharing stories of readers' experiences in order to inspire, inform, and motivate others. A website has been created at www.eightshifts.com where I will post readers' stories and their experiences with the material in the book. You can visit the website to see how others have applied the eight shifts. You can also share your own experiences in the name of partnership with and service to others by sending me your story. E-mail it to comments@eightshifts.com or visit the www.eightshifts.com website and enter the information via the form you will find there. You may also mail your story to me at the publisher address listed at the front of the book.

Please provide your city and state, or country if located outside the U.S. The website postings will not use names. Even if you don't want your experiences posted on the website, I'm interested in hearing how the book has impacted your life.

One last item . . .

In honor of the ancestors and for the sake of the next generations, I ask you, the reader, the following three questions:

1. Will you implement ideas, practices or concepts to improve your own health, wellness and well-being?

2. Will you be of service by implementing ideas, practices or concepts to improve the health, wellness and well-being of someone else?

3. Will you share the information in this book with at least one other person to give them the opportunity to enhance their own health, wellness and well-being?

YES – YES – YES – NOW

Eight Shifts - REAC LPPS

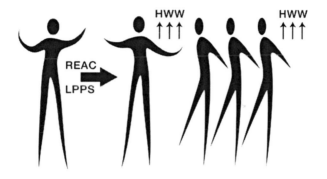

Eight Shifts - REAC LPPS

Reframing

Empowerment

Awakening

Choices

Eight Shifts - REAC LPPS

Living

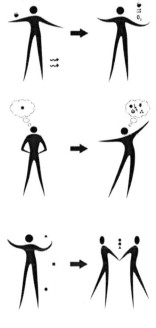

Possibilities

Partnership

Service

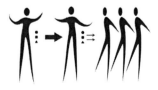

Eight Shifts - REAC LPPS

Reframing
Wellness vs Health
Mind and Body

Living
Movement and Exercise
Breathing
Sleep and Rest
Food and Wellness

Empowerment
Role of the Individual
Choosing Empowerment

Possibilities
Wellness Modalities
Acupuncture
Herbs

Awakening
Your Body as Teacher
Heeding the "Warning Lights"

Partnership
Healing Presence
Language as "Treatment"
The Yin Yang of Relationships

Choices
The Observer
Phenomena vs Story
Small Mind, Large Mind
Upset Is Optional
Yes, Yes, Now
Addressing Stress

Service
You Are a Leader
Seven Generations
Power to Make an Impact

The Guarantee

CHAPTER 11

THE GUARANTEE

Eight Shifts for Wellness comes with a guarantee. I genuinely be-lieve the information I am attempting to explain and illustrate can help every single person make a positive impact on their life and a positive impact on the life of someone else.

I have not done a successful job in writing the book if you read it and do not discover (1) one idea, concept, practice, or tool you can use to enhance your health, wellness, or well-being, and (2) one idea, concept, practice, or tool you can use to enhance the health, wellness, or well-being of someone else.

If you have not discovered these two golden nuggets, please e-mail me at marc@eightshifts.com or write to me at the publisher's address in the front of the book. I will e-mail or write you to clarify and expand on the material and assist you in uncovering your golden nuggets.

This is not the end.

It's a beginning!

I invite you to make a shift for the sake of

→ Yourself

→ Your family

→ Loved ones

→ Others

→ Future generations

Notes

INTRODUCTION

1. The Tai Sophia Institute (www.tai.edu), located in Howard County, Maryland, was founded by Robert Duggan and Dianne Connelly and has grown into a premier accredited graduate school focused on health and wellness. This dynamic school which is anchored in the modern world and respects ancient healing traditions has an expanding offering of wellness-based academic programs. Programs offered by the Tai Sophia Institute as of spring 2011 include masters' degrees in acupuncture, nutrition and integrative health, herbal medicine, and transformative leadership and social change. Graduate certificate programs include wellness coaching, health coaching, medical herbalism, herbal studies, Chinese herbs, and transformative leadership. The Institute's twelve-acre campus includes a natural care center where practitioners offer wellness services; a café, bookstore, and extensive library focused on wellness and well-being; an herbal dispensary; and an herbal garden. The Institute's faculty, students, and staff provide voluntary service to the community. Representatives of the Institute have testified before Congress on wellness topics and served on the White House Commission on Complementary and Alternative Medicine. In addition, the Institute has hosted symposiums, seminars, and conferences on

wellness, and members of its faculty have conducted workshops around the world. The school's name derives from the Chinese word *tai*, which means "great," and the Greek word *sophia*, which means "wisdom."

2. James Fries et al., "Reducing Health Care Costs by Reducing the Need and Demand for Medical Services," *New England Journal of Medicine*, July 29, 1993.

3. Deepak Chopra et al., "Alternative Medicine Is Mainstream," opinion article in *The Wall Street Journal*, January 9, 2009.

CHAPTER 1 – SHIFT 1: REFRAMING

1. World Health Organization, "Frequently asked questions," http://who.int/suggestions/faq/en/ (accessed October 24, 2009).

2. National Wellness Institute, "Defining Wellness," http://www.nationalwellness.org/index.php?id_tier=2&id_c=26 (accessed October 15, 2009).

3. Lin Yutang, *The Wisdom of China and India* (New York: The Modern Library, 1942), 1064. By permission of Richard Ming Lai and Hsiang Jo Lin.

CHAPTER 2 – SHIFT 2: EMPOWERMENT

1. Anees Sheikh and Katharina Sheikh, *Healing East and West: Ancient Wisdom and Modern Psychology* (New York: Wiley, 1965), 66-67.

2. Elliott Dacher, "At the Heart of the New Medicine," *Meridians*, Autumn 1998, 20.

3. Roger Jahnke, *The Healer Within* (San Francisco: HarperCollins, 1997), 4.

4. Elliott Dacher, "At the Heart of the New Medicine," *Meridians,* Autumn 1998, 20.

5. John Sullivan, *Living Large: Transformative Work at the Inter-section of Ethics and Spirituality* (Laurel, MD: Tai Sophia Press, 2004), 27-28.

CHAPTER 3 - SHIFT 3: AWAKENING

1. The concept "Your body is wise" was first taught to me by Robert Duggan, President Emeritus, co-founder and faculty member of the Tai Sophia Institute. Mr. Duggan, MA, MAc(UK), has been a practitioner of traditional acupuncture since 1973 and is the author of *Common Sense for the Healing Arts.*

2. Lin Yutang, *The Wisdom of China and India* (New York: The Modern Library, 1942), 1064. By permission of Richard Ming Lai and Hsiang Jo Lin.

CHAPTER 4 - SHIFT 4: CHOICES

1. The expression "Create a story big enough to live in" is used at the Tai Sophia Institute as part of the teaching of phenomena and story.

2. This section is based on the work of John Sullivan, PhD, includ-ing his book *Living Large: Transformative Work at the Intersec-tion of Ethics and Spirituality* and work he has done for the Tai Sophia Institute in designing its Masters of Arts in Transforma-tive Leadership and Social Change program. The four-line quote is taught at the Tai Sophia Institute. Dr. Sullivan is Maude Sharpe Powell Professor of Philosophy Emeritus and Distinguished Uni-versity Professor Emeritus at Elon University in North Carolina.

He is the author of *To Come to Life More Fully*; *Living Large: Transformative Work at the Intersection of Ethics and Spirituality*; *The Spiral of Seasons: Welcoming the Gifts of Later Life*; and *The Fourfold Path to Wholeness: A Compass for the Heart*.

3. The expression "Upset is optional" was first taught to me by Robert Duggan. It is a popular saying at the Tai Sophia Institute and some people have it printed on bumper stickers or engraved on stones they display on a desk or table as a reminder of the principle.

4. The exercise "Yes, Yes, Now" was first taught to me by Dianne Connelly, Chancellor Emeritus, co-founder and faculty member of the Tai Sophia Institute. Dr. Connelly, PhD, MAc(UK), MA, has been a practitioner of traditional acupuncture since 1973 and is the author of *Traditional Acupuncture: The Law of the Five Elements*; *All Sickness Is Homesickness*; and *Medicine Words: Language of Love for the Treatment Room of Life*. She is the co-author of *Alive and Awake: Wisdom for Kids*.

5. Excellent resources for information on stress are: The American Institute of Stress, http://www.stress.org; and Robert Sapolsky, *Why Zebras Don't Get Ulcers: An Updated Guide to Stress, Stress-Related Diseases, and Coping* (New York: W. H. Freeman and Company, 1998).

6. Roger Darlington's World, "Stories to Make You Think," 'The Wise Teacher and the Jar,' http://www.rogerdarlington.co.uk/stories.html (accessed October 29, 2009).

CHAPTER 5 – SHIFT 5: LIVING

1. World Health Organization, "Global Strategy on Diet, Physical Activity and Health," http://www.who.int/dietphysicalactivity/

en (accessed October 24, 2009).

2. National Center for Complementary and Alternative Medicine, National Institute of Health, "Yoga for Health: An Introduction," http://nccam.nih.gov/health/yoga/introduction.htm (accessed February 1, 2010).

3. Roger Jahnke, *The Healer Within* (San Francisco: HarperCollins, 1997), 84.

4. Ibid.

5. Ibid., 86.

6. Ibid.

7. National Sleep Foundation, "Let Sleep Work for You," http://www.sleepfoundation.org/let-sleep-work-you (accessed October 16, 2009).

8. Robert Duggan, *Common Sense for the Healing Arts* (Laurel, MD: Tai Sophia Press, 2003), 33-34.

9. National Sleep Foundation, "Sleep-Wake Cycle: Its Physiology and Impact on Health," http://www.sleepfoundation.org (accessed October 16, 2009).

10. Michael Pollan, *In Defense of Food* (New York: Penguin Books, 2008), 90.

11. World Health Organization. "Global Strategy on Diet, Physical Activity and Health," http://www.who.int/dietphysicalactivity/publications/facts/cancer/en/ (accessed October 24, 2009).

12. Michael Pollan, *In Defense of Food* (New York: Penguin Books, 2008), 164.

13. Ibid., 136.

14. Annemarie Colbin, "Why Should We Eat Whole Foods?," http://www.foodandhealing.com/articles/article-wholefoods.htm (accessed October 27, 2009).

15. Ibid.

16. Mark Hyman, "Eating Medicine: Food as Pharmacology," *Alternative Therapies in Health and Medicine*, Nov/Dec 2005, 2.

17. John Sullivan, *Living Large: Transformative Work at the Intersection of Ethics and Spirituality* (Laurel, MD: Tai Sophia Press, 2004), 167-168.

18. Nicholas Albery et al., *The Book of Inspirations: A Directory of Social Inventions* (London: The Institute for Social Inventions, 2000), 48.

CHAPTER 6 - SHIFT 6: POSSIBILITIES

1. Excellent resources for information on the Flexner Report are: Robert Bowman, "Flexner's Impact on American Medicine," http://www.ruralmedicaleducation.org/flexner.htm (accessed February 18, 2011); and Mark Hiatt and Christopher Stockton, "The Impact of the Flexner Report on the Fate of Medical Schools in North America after 1909," *Journal of American Physicians and Surgeons*, Summer 2003, 37-40.

2. National Center for Complementary and Alternative Medicine, National Institute of Health, "Acupuncture: An Introduction," http://nccam.nih.gov/health/acupuncture/introduction.htm (accessed February 1, 2010).

3. National Center for Complementary and Alternative Medicine, National Institute of Health, "Ayurvedic Medicine: An Introduction," http://nccam.nih.gov/health/ayurveda/introduction.htm (accessed February 1, 2010).

4. National Center for Complementary and Alternative Medicine, National Institute of Health, "Chiropractic: An Introduction," http://nccam.nih.gov/health/chiropractic/ (accessed February

1, 2010).

5. Associated Bodywork and Massage Professionals, "Glossary: Types of Massage and Bodywork Defined," http://www.massage-therapy.com/glossary/index.php (accessed December 18, 2009).

6. National Center for Complementary and Alternative Medicine, National Institute of Health, "Homeopathy: An Introduction," http://nccam.nih.gov/health/homeopathy/ (accessed February 1, 2010).

7. National Center for Complementary and Alternative Medicine, National Institute of Health, "Massage Therapy: An Introduction," http://nccam.nih.gov/health/massage/ (accessed February 1, 2010).

8. National Center for Complementary and Alternative Medicine, National Institute of Health, "Meditation: An Introduction," http://nccam.nih.gov/health/meditation/overview.htm (accessed February 1, 2010).

9. National Center for Complementary and Alternative Medicine, National Institute of Health, "An Introduction to Naturopathy," http://nccam.nih.gov/health/naturopathy/ (accessed February 1, 2010).

10. American Osteopathic Association, http://www.osteopathic.org (accessed December 18, 2009).

11. Associated Bodywork and Massage Professionals, "Glossary: Types of Massage and Bodywork Defined," http://www.massage-therapy.com/glossary/index.php (accessed December 18, 2009).

12. National Center for Complementary and Alternative Medicine, National Institute of Health, "Reiki: An Introduction," http://nccam.nih.gov/health/reiki/ (accessed February 1, 2010).

13. National Center for Complementary and Alternative Medicine,

National Institute of Health, "Tai Chi: An Introduction," http://nccam.nih.gov/health/taichi/ (accessed February 1, 2010).

14. National Center for Complementary and Alternative Medicine, National Institute of Health, "Yoga for Health: An Introduction," http://nccam.nih.gov/health/yoga/introduction.htm (accessed February 1, 2010).

15. Zero Balancing Health Association, http://www.zerobalancing.com (accessed November 25, 2009).

16. Dianne Connelly, *Traditional Acupuncture: The Law of the Five Elements* (Laurel, MD: Tai Sophia Institute, 1994), 3-4.

17. Ibid., 89-100.

18. Simon Mills, *The Essential Book of Herbal Medicine* (London: Arkana, 1993), 148-150. Simon Mills, MA, FNIMH, MCPP, based in the United Kingdom, is the founder of the herbal medicine program at the Tai Sophia Institute and a faculty member in the program. He is a world-renowned expert and author in the field of herbalism.

19. Simon Mills, *The Essential Book of Herbal Medicine* (London: Arkana, 1993), 150.

20. Ibid., 4.

21. World Health Organization, "Traditional Medicine," http://www.who.int/mediacentre/factsheets/fs134/en/index/html (accessed October 24, 2009).

22. Simon Mills, *The Essential Book of Herbal Medicine* (London: Arkana, 1993), 7-10.

23. Ibid., 8.

24. Ibid., 23.

25. Ibid., 7.

26. John Sullivan, *Living Large: Transformative Work at the Inter-*

section of Ethics and Spirituality (Laurel, MD: Tai Sophia Press, 2004), 35.

CHAPTER 7 – SHIFT 7: PARTNERSHIP

1. The concept of "being a healing presence" is taught at the Tai Sophia Institute. The material is this section reflects my interpretation of this concept and the concept of being a wellness practitioner.

2. Resources on yin and yang include: Dianne Connelly, *Traditional Acupuncture: The Law of the Five Elements* (Laurel, MD: Tai Sophia Institute, 1994), 13-14; and John Sullivan, *Living Large: Transformative Work at the Intersection of Ethics and Spirituality* (Laurel, MD: Tai Sophia Press, 2004), 76-77.

3. Discussion of relationships includes concepts by John Sullivan, including material in his book *Living Large: Transformative Work at the Intersection of Ethics and Spirituality* (Laurel, MD: Tai Sophia Press, 2004), 132-137.

4. *Spiritual Stories and Parables*, "Losing Everything," http://www.spiritual-short-stories.com/spiritual-short-story-201-losing+everything.html (accessed February 18, 2011).

CHAPTER 8 – SHIFT 8: SERVICE

1. The expression and concept "lead from any seat" is based on "leading from any chair" in *The Art of Possibility: Transforming Professional and Personal Life* by Rosamund Stone Zander and Benjamin Zander (Boston: Harvard Business School Press, 2000), 67-77.

2. John Sullivan, *Living Large: Transformative Work at the Inter-

section of Ethics and Spirituality (Laurel, MD: Tai Sophia Press, 2004), 102.

3. Robert Duggan, *Common Sense for the Healing Arts* (Laurel, MD: Tai Sophia Press, 2003), 42.

4. Rosamund Stone Zander and Benjamin Zander, *The Art of Possibility: Transforming Professional and Personal Life* (Boston: Harvard Business Press, 2000), 55.

5. Roger Darlington's World, "Stories to Make You Think," 'Chopsticks," http://www.rogerdarlington.co.uk/stories.html (accessed October 29, 2009).

CHAPTER 9 – PRACTICES

1. The term and concept of "being a beginner" rather than thinking of something as being hard was first taught to me by Dianne Connelly.

Bibliography

Albery, Nicholas, et al. *The Book of Inspirations: A Directory of Social Inventions.* London: The Institute for Social Inventions, 2000.

American Institute of Stress. http://www.stress.org.

American Osteopathic Association. http://www.osteopathic.org.

Associated Bodywork and Massage Professionals. http://www.massagetherapy.com.

Bowman, Robert. "Flexner's Impact on American Medicine." http://www.ruralmedicaleducation.org/flexner.htm.

Chopra, Deepak, et al. "Alternative Medicine Is Mainstream." Opinion article in *The Wall Street Journal*, January 9, 2009.

Colbin, Annemarie. "Why Should We Eat Whole Foods?" http://www.foodandhealing.com/articles/article-wholefoods.htm.

Connelly, Dianne. *Traditional Acupuncture: The Law of the Five Elements.* Laurel, MD: Tai Sophia Institute, 1994.

Dacher, Elliott. "At the Heart of the New Medicine." *Meridians,* Autumn 1998.

Duggan, Robert. *Common Sense for the Healing Arts.* Laurel, MD: Tai Sophia Press, 2003.

Fries, James, et al. "Reducing Health Care Costs by Reducing the Need and Demand for Medical Services." *New England Journal of Medicine,* July 29, 1993.

Hiatt, Mark and Christopher Stockton. "The Impact of the

Flexner Report on the Fate of Medical Schools in North America after 1909." *Journal of American Physicians and Surgeons*, Summer 2003.

Hyman, Mark. "Eating Medicine: Food as Pharmacology." *Alternative Therapies in Health and Medicine*, Nov/Dec 2005.

Jahnke, Roger. *The Healer Within*. San Francisco: HarperCollins, 1997.

Mills, Simon. *The Essential Book of Herbal Medicine*. London: Arkana, 1993.

National Center for Complementary and Alternative Medicine, National Institute of Health. http://nccam.nih.gov.

National Sleep Foundation. http://www.sleepfoundation.org.

National Wellness Institute. http://www.nationalwellness.org.

Pollan, Michael. *In Defense of Food*. New York: Penguin Books, 2008.

Roger Darlington's World. "Stories to Make You Think." http://www.rogerdarlington.co.uk.

Sapolsky, Robert. *Why Zebras Don't Get Ulcers: An Updated Guide to Stress, Stress-Related Diseases, and Coping*. New York: W. H. Freeman, 1998.

Sheikh, Anees and Katharina Sheikh. *Healing East and West: Ancient Wisdom and Modern Psychology*. New York: Wiley, 1989.

Spiritual Short Stories. http://www.spiritual-short-stories.com.

Sullivan, John. *Living Large: Transformative Work at the Intersection of Ethics and Spirituality*. Laurel, MD: Tai Sophia Press, 2004.

Tai Sophia Institute. http://www.tai.edu.

World Health Organization. http://www.who.int.

Yutang, Lin. *The Wisdom of China and India*. New York: The

Modern Library, 1942.

Zander, Rosamund Stone and Benjamin Zander. *The Art of Possibility: Transforming Professional and Personal Life.* Boston: Harvard Business Press, 2000.

Zero Balancing Health Association. http://www.zerobalancing.com.

Acknowledgments

F irst I want to thank my wife Kim and children Jason, Megan, and Alex for their love, support, and what they have taught me about life. Someone mentioned to me that writing this book is a major accomplishment and I should feel proud. Although I am proud of the book and the potential it has to make a difference in the lives of many people, the proudest aspect of my life is my children. They are grounded, mature, well-rounded individuals of whom a father and mother could not be prouder. Kim deserves most of the credit for this outcome, and the kids and I are fortunate to have her in our lives.

The book was inspired by the information, knowledge, and wisdom that I was first exposed to at the Tai Sophia Institute. I want to thank my amazing teachers in the Transformative Leadership and Social Change master's program and all my classmates from that program and from the Transformative Leadership graduate certificate program. Learning takes place not just from the teachers but also from other students who are filled with unbelievable insight, caring, compassion and a commitment to use what they have learned to have a positive impact on the world.

I also want to thank my colleagues, the staff at the Tai Sophia Institute—hard-working dedicated people who recognize they are working for an organization that is having an important impact in the world.

Working and spending most of my waking hours with this group of people has been a pleasure.

There are certain individuals who are part of the Tai Sophia community who read early drafts and provided valuable input and feedback. Thank you, Guy Hollyday, Pam Fleming, Robert Duggan, Susan Duggan, Dianne Connelly, John Sullivan, Judi Broida, Mary Ellen Zorbaugh, and Jeff Millison. I also received invaluable input, advice and encouragement from two people in the publishing industry. Rudy Schur and Regina Sara Ryan, I cannot thank you enough for your generosity and willingness to share your publishing wisdom with me. To all of you, I say you are great examples of partnership and service. Each of you graciously spent time and energy to assist me, and as a result you are helping every reader of the book, and through the readers you are helping every person they in turn help.

I was extremely fortunate to work with an editor who is quite frankly awesome. Thank you, Nancy Lewis, for your commitment to the vision and for using your incredible talents to help create a book that will make a difference.

Just as awesome is my book designer, Brion Sausser. Thank you, Brion, for blending your creative talents with my abstract guidance to create a cover and book that reflects the vision and is worthy of the importance of the topic.

I am very aware that in writing this book I am the messenger standing on the shoulders of legions of others, just as Tai Sophia stands on the shoulders of the teachers and wisdom leaders who came before it. I want to acknowledge and thank everyone who has been part of the Tai Sophia community for their unique contributions and support of such a worthy endeavor. Bob and Dianne, thank you for founding this extraordinary organization. My appreciation goes as well to the Board of Trustees, staff, faculty, students, practitioners, patients, donors, lenders, participants in community programs, guest speakers, and others who have been part of this community. Thank you all. Last, I acknowledge with gratitude the teachers, practitioners, and individuals who for generations have been passing on their knowledge and wisdom about health and wellness for the sake of others.

About the Author

Marc Levin has a graduate certificate in Transformative Leadership from the Tai Sophia Institute (www.tai.edu), an accredited graduate school focused on health and wellness, and an MBA and a BS in accounting from the University of Maryland. He is in the final stages of earning a master's degree in Transformative Leadership and Social Change from the Tai Sophia Institute, and is a certified public accountant. Mr. Levin and his family are volunteer puppy raisers for Canine Companions for Independence (www.cci.org), a nonprofit organization that provides trained dogs to children and adults with disabilities, free of charge. He has three grown children and lives with his wife in Maryland.

Learn more about Marc Levin and the eight shifts at
WWW.EIGHTSHIFTS.COM.

New Possibilities Await You!

CPSIA information can be obtained at www.ICGtesting.com
Printed in the USA
266151BV00002B/1/P